the **youth** equation

the **youth** equation

Take **10** Years Off Your Face

Jeffrey S. Dover, M.D.

with Cara Birnbaum

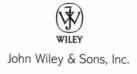

WILEY

John Wiley & Sons, Inc.

Published by John Wiley & Sons, Inc., Hoboken, New Jersey
Published simultaneously in Canada

Library of Congress Cataloging-in-Publication Data:

Dover, Jeffrey S.
  The youth equation : take 10 years off your face / Jeffrey Dover with Cara Birnbaum.
    p. cm.
  Includes bibliographical references and index.
  ISBN 978-0-470-19180-4 (cloth)
  1. Skin-care and hygiene. 2. Rejuvenation. 3. Beauty, Personal. 4. Women—Health and hygiene. 5. Dermatology—Popular works. I. Birnbaum, Cara. II. Title.
  RL87.D68 2009
  646.7'26—dc22   2008041535

Printed in the United States of America

10 9 8 7 6 5 4 3 2 1

For Isabel and Sophie
and
for Tania

Contents

Acknowledgments   ix

Introduction   1

Part One **The Equation**   **9**

    1 Your Skin's Virtual Age Quiz   1 1

    2 Skin Deep   15

    3 Cleanse   35

    4 Treat   51

    5 Prevent   95

Part Two **The Prescription**   **113**

    6 No Surgery, No Kidding: Dr. Dover's
      Six-Week Plan for Younger-Looking Skin   115

Part Three **Beyond Topicals**   **153**

    7 Injection Options   155

    8 Lasers and Light Options   191

    9 Surgical Cosmetic Procedures   223

    Glossary   245

    Index   263

Acknowledgments

Tremendous effort went into this book, and there are many friends and colleagues who helped along the way.

Thanks to Deb Maue, who first suggested that I write a book on skin care for my patients and the public, and to Carl Schmitt, who took over from Deb. He saw the value and importance of *The Youth Equation* and encouraged me to stay the course.

Thanks to my agents, Jill Kneerim and Brettne Bloom, without whose advice, guidance, and tenacity the book would never have found life.

I'm very grateful to our editor, Tom Miller, who offered us the opportunity to publish *The Youth Equation*. His years of editorial expertise proved invaluable for refining our ideas and concepts.

For making those ideas and concepts more than just words on a page, I thank our illustrator, Leigh Campbell, who turned my abstract sketches into beautiful drawings. Lou Frisina and Dr. A. Jay Burns supplied me with terrific before-and-after photos of their patients.

Dr. Ken Arndt, my mentor and close friend, has been a constant source of motivation and encouragement. His steadfast curiosity, judgment, encouragement, and generosity have helped shape who I am as a doctor—and as an author.

My wife and dermatology colleague, Dr. Tania Phillips, has been a never-ending inspiration. I thank her for continuous encouragement, ideas, guidance and thoughts, for repeatedly reading through early drafts, and for fine-tuning the final manuscript.

Last and most important, I would like to thank my coauthor, Cara Birnbaum, without whose indefatigable energy and even temperament this project would never have been completed. Despite many sleepless nights (Cara's first child, June, was born while we were writing the book), her dedication to the project never wavered.

Introduction

Denise looked worried when she walked into my office for the first time. She was preoccupied with the fine lines, wrinkles, and brown spots that had started to emerge on her face. Denise, a very attractive local philanthropist with chestnut-colored hair who was wearing large designer sunglasses and an exquisite outfit, was in her late thirties, and those early signs of aging were fairly normal. Nevertheless, Denise was willing to do anything and everything in her power to try to reverse the clock. She asked me about Botox and lasers and cosmetic surgery. During the visit she pulled a weird electrical muscle-stimulating device out of her purse—a gadget she had bought on a television shopping channel that was supposed to erase her wrinkles. She had the good sense to ask me about it before using it on her face, and I asked her if I could hold on to it. I keep it in my top desk drawer, as a funny and poignant reminder of the things that people will do to look younger.

People are paying more attention than ever to the appearance of their skin, especially to how young or how old their skin looks. You should see my appointment book. It's filled with the names of patients who travel from near and far to my Boston office. Some come specifically to inquire about ways to slow or reverse the aging process. Others come for general dermatology issues, such as eczema, acne, melasma, or skin cancer, yet they, too, very frequently (often just before leaving the examination room) bring up their crow's feet, frown lines, wrinkles, or brown spots, or ask me why their skin doesn't have quite the youthful glow it did five years ago.

This brings us to the good news: my patients are so aware of each little spot, line, and wrinkle because of all the tools we now have to erase them. You can't go anywhere today without passing a department store or a drugstore display for a so-called miracle anti-aging cream, reading about a fancy new laser that promises to make you look ten years younger with one treatment during your lunch hour, or seeing a glossy magazine ad for Botox and cosmetic fillers like Restylane and Juvederm. My patients are flooded with so much information about the latest anti-aging skin-care products that by the time they get to my office, some of them are telling *me* what to prescribe.

Sometimes they're right on target. Sometimes they're not. With all of the articles, ads, and sound bites floating around skin-care circles these days, it's hard to know which products and treatments really live up to their promises—and for those that do, which ones are right for any given skin type. Given all the treatment options available, it's even harder to avoid becoming obsessed with every line, brown spot, broken blood vessel, or wrinkle. Not long ago, one of my patients—a well-known TV personality who was watched by millions of people every day—actually brought in a *suitcase* of products she used to clean, tone, and exfoliate her face raw. She was beside herself about the wrinkles under her eyes. It turned out that she had eczema, which was drying out her skin and making those wrinkles more visible—and her giant suitcase full of products was only making matters worse.

Pretty scary, right? Caring for your complexion should never be about attacking it, even if you are declaring war on those crow's feet and wrinkles. Real improvement starts when you pause to listen to your skin. Invest in the right cleansers, moisturizers, creams, and lotions, and they will pay you back. Your skin will look brighter, younger, and more beautiful than you ever thought possible. As for more aggressive procedures, like Botox, lasers, and fillers, they've evolved so that they brighten, smooth, and firm the skin and even out its color without making you look like a statue from Madame Tussauds wax museum. In my opinion, the best anti-aging treatments, whether they come from a serum or a syringe, a laser or a cream, don't offer a tight, pulled-back, extreme makeover. Instead, they leave you looking like a more refreshed, relaxed, youthful version of yourself.

In addition, any good skin-care regimen should be easy, pampering, and, dare I say, sort of fun. These days, you can find potent, effective products at the local drugstore—products that feel amazing going on and that smell like the products used at a high-end day spa. As for those minimally invasive in-office procedures, most really *can* be done during your lunch hour—in much less time than it takes to have your hair highlighted.

So here's the $64,000 question: With the wealth of anti-aging treatments out there, how do you know which ones will actually turn back the clock for your skin? The simple answer is that you don't—not from a cursory glance at the label, anyway. Every so-called miracle cream in the beauty aisle might *claim* that it's best for you, but think about it: the people who printed that on the box don't know whether you're a twenty-year-old college junior or a sixty-five-year-old grandmother. They don't know whether you spent your teen years baking on the beach or battling acne—or both. So, as enticing as those promises are, you have to take them with a serious grain of salt.

The secret to finding the products and procedures that truly will stop and reverse the signs of aging in your skin is understanding exactly how old your complexion is right now. You might be thinking, *I'm aware of how old I am—painfully aware.* However, there's a big difference between your actual age and your skin's virtual age, a number I call SVA. I determine a patient's SVA using the following three basic factors:

1. **Lifestyle.** Do you smoke? Eat a balanced diet? Wear sunscreen? What is your skin-care regimen like?

2. **Family history.** How old were your mother and your father when they saw their first wrinkles? How does your parents' skin look now?

3. **Current appearance.** Do you have any fine lines? Does your skin sag? Is your pigmentation uneven?

No one likes thinking about the age of her skin. Nevertheless, consider this: once you know your SVA, you're already ahead of the game, because you can use your score to determine exactly how your skin is doing and how to turn back the clock, starting right now. I've devised a multipronged but simple anti-aging plan that's perfectly tailored to the current state, or SVA, of your complexion. In many cases, the plan is so straightforward that my patients can take it right to the local drugstore, navigate their way through the baffling skin-care aisle, and walk out with exactly the few products they need to produce the kind of smooth, radiant skin they haven't seen in years. In fact, if you follow my plan diligently (no cheating—no matter how tired you are) for six weeks, you can easily knock a few years off your SVA. Stick with the program, and the improvement will only continue.

My plan is straightforward but incredibly effective. Anyone who glances at the patients in our waiting room will see that it works. Of course, I hardly expect you to trek out to our Boston office for your SVA score and a coordinating treatment plan. This book contains everything you need to calculate that number on your own and to write your own personalized prescription for a younger, healthier-looking complexion. Skip ahead a few pages, and you'll find a short quiz I developed that will tell you how old your skin looks and behaves. Once you've determined your SVA, you might want to go directly to the chapters that detail my decade-by-decade "cleanse—treat—prevent" formula that will make your skin look smoother, firmer, and more lustrous within weeks, without procedures or surgery.

To truly reap the benefits of this book, however, I urge you to start at the beginning. Chapter 2 offers the complete lowdown on how and why the skin ages. The next three chapters outline everything you need to know about the lotions and potions that actually live up to their promises—from cleansers that brighten the skin to serums that reduce sun damage and fight acne. I follow that with a six-week plan, customized to your SVA, that will make big changes with only a handful of products. Because some people want to supplement those topical treatments with more aggressive treatments, the second half of the book covers in-office procedures like Botox, cosmetic fillers, light-source devices, and even plastic surgery. I've packed each chapter with the kind of no-nonsense, cutting-edge information that I give my own patients, along with simple equations that explain exactly what you need in order to encourage your skin to begin "acting" and *looking* younger.

A few words about products: as I've said earlier—and will continue to repeat—you do *not* have to take out a second mortgage to afford an excellent skin-care regimen. These days, any high-quality drugstore carries not only great anti-aging prescription topical creams, like retinoids and antibiotic lotions, but also a wide selection of effective, well-made over-the-counter products that impress even the most experienced dermatologists (like me). I'll admit, I have a favorite: Skin Effects, my own line, which is sold exclusively through CVS Pharmacy nationwide. Many of my patients are the kind of people who like to buy high-end, top-quality products—at great prices. So I developed this line for them. I've spent years creating potent antiwrinkle creams, soufflé-like moisturizers, and powerful, broad-spectrum sunscreens—most of which cost less than twenty dollars—by using the best ingredients money can buy and working with the very same laboratories used by many of the A-list skin-care companies that charge hundreds of dollars an ounce for their potions.

Enough about Skin Effects. My point is: don't judge a skin-care product based on its fancy price, packaging, or glossy ads, or by the fact that it's sold at an expensive department-store counter. You can find amazing creams, cleansers, and sunscreens wherever you shop. The key is knowing what to look for. That means searching for the right ingredients as well as for the right brands and products. You'll notice that I make specific product recommendations throughout this book. I divide them into three categories: drugstore, department store, and lines that are available only in doctors' offices. Keep in mind that you can find many of these brands online if you plug the names into a search engine.

I am partial to certain products. These include several national brands that are available at the drugstore. Olay offers products with retinol, peptides, and other ingredients that you'll read about later. You really can't go wrong with anything made by Neutrogena, Pond's, Aveeno, and L'Oreal. These are huge companies with even bigger reputations, so you'd never catch them launching a product that wasn't just as effective as its department-store counterpart—but far more affordable. (If you happen not to agree, most drugstores will let you bring your products back for a full refund.)

Of course, I do have patients who swear by their $200 jar of beautifully packaged cream. I certainly don't argue with them, because department stores and beauty specialty shops like Sephora carry a range of lines that are as effective as they are luxurious. So if you really want to pamper yourself, you might consider brands like La Prairie, Orlane, Cle de Peau, Sisley, SkinCeuticals, Dr. Brandt, DDF, Murad, Patricia Wexler M.D. Dermatology, and N.V. Perricone M.D.

As for lines that are offered only through doctors' offices, I love SkinCare Prescription, which my dermatology colleagues at our practice, SkinCare Physicians, created after years of effort. I also like Prevage, the TNS Recovery Complex line of growth-factor products made by SkinMedica and NeoStrata, among others.

Please remember that the product recommendations I sprinkle throughout the first half of this book are not an exhaustive list. Naming all my favorites would require its own separate book. I'm merely offering a sampling of the great skin-care products that are available right now. Also, keep in mind that skin-care companies change the names of their products frequently, so if you can't track down the exact name of a cleanser, cream, or sunscreen on one of my lists, you should be able to find something very similar by the same brand.

One thing you won't read much about in this book is miraculous, overnight results. I don't believe in sending people on wild-goose chases for trendy youth serums that cost $500 or more a bottle. Unfortunately, the vast majority of those really expensive products don't come close to delivering; if they did, I'd be using them, and so would other dermatologists! Here's what you can expect to find in this book: the ingredients and products that will make you look significantly better in six weeks—and worlds better after six months. I promise that these are products that won't leave you bankrupt. You'll also learn which in-office procedures are worth the time and the money. In short, this book offers a comprehensive anti-aging prescription. Nobody but you has to know how old your skin really is.

the equation

Cleanse, treat, prevent. The concept sounds simple, but you'd be amazed at how many people have trouble actually putting it into practice. Maybe you're one of them. You might think your skin looks young enough to excuse you from performing all three steps day and night. You might think you're too busy. Or, most likely, when it comes to finding the products you need, you might be so overwhelmed by the sheer selection in the drugstore or the department store that you wind up throwing your hands in the air and walking out the door. In part one, I'll dispense with the confusion by first determining what type of skin you have. Then, I'll walk you through my "cleanse, treat, prevent" regimen and show you why no one can afford to skip a single step.

Your Skin's Virtual Age Quiz

Before you turn another page of this book, I want you to stop and take a short quiz. These are the questions I ask my own patients when they walk into my office. You won't have to open any books to find the answers or think for more than a moment about each one. There's no right or wrong answer. However, for such a simple quiz, it offers profound benefits. In less than three minutes, you'll know your skin's virtual age, or SVA. This is your tool for beginning to piece together your personalized anti-aging prescription—and start changing the face you see in the mirror every morning.

Directions: Write down your actual age, then add and subtract points according to your answers to the questions that follow.

My actual age is: _____

Lifestyle

1. I wear sunscreen
   A. Every day of the year (subtract 1)
   B. Sometimes (during the summer, on sunny days, or when I plan to be outside for several hours) (add 0)
   C. Very rarely (add 1)

2. As a child, how many of your summer days were spent outside?
   A. Few (subtract 1)
   B. Some (add 0)
   C. As many as possible (add 1)

3. When I was a teenager, sun exposure was something
   A. I avoided (subtract 1)
   B. I didn't think about much (add 0)
   C. I tried to get as often as possible (add 1)

4. Did you ever smoke?
   A. Never (add 0)
   B. I used to smoke, but I stopped more than ten years ago (add 0)
   C. I used to smoke, but I stopped less than ten years ago (add 1)
   D. Yes, and I still do (add 2)

5. I eat several servings of fruits and vegetables
   A. Every day (subtract 1)
   B. Once a week (add 0)
   C. Do French fries and ketchup count? (add 1)

6. I exercise
   A. Three times a week or more (subtract 1)
   B. Once a week (add 0)
   C. As little as possible (add 1)

If your parents are living, answer the next two questions. If not, skip to question 9.

Genes

7. Right now, my mother
   A. Looks younger than her age (subtract 1)
   B. Looks about her age (add 0)
   C. Might be mistaken for my grandmother (add 1)

8. Right now, my father
   A. Looks younger than his age (subtract 1)
   B. Looks about his age (add 0)
   C. Might be mistaken for my grandfather (add 1)

Current Appearance

Take out a hand mirror and stand near a bright window or in your brightly lit bathroom. (Don't be scared!)

9. The lines on the sides of my eyes are
   A. Pretty much nonexistent, even when I smile or frown (subtract 1)
   B. Apparent only when I smile or frown (add 0)
   C. Quite visible, regardless of my expression (add 1)

10. The lines and crinkles under my eyes are
    A. Very faint and few in number (subtract 1)
    B. Noticeable and bothersome (add 0)
    C. Deep and numerous (add 1)

11. When I lift my eyebrows and then release them, any forehead lines
    A. Vanish immediately (subtract 1)
    B. Take a second or two to fade (add 0)
    C. Stick around (add 1)

12. My general skin tone and color is
    A. Even (subtract 1)
    B. Slightly blotchy in certain areas, such as my cheeks (add 0)
    C. Uneven, with brown spots scattered around my face (add 1)

13. When I touch the skin under my jawline along my upper neck, it feels
    A. Supple and firm (subtract 1)
    B. A bit more jiggly than it used to (add 0)
    C. Saggy and loose (add 1)

My skin's virtual age is: actual age + (or –) test score = _____

Please don't be discouraged if your SVA is higher than your actual age. This doesn't mean that you're too far gone or that your wrinkles and brown spots will only get worse. On the contrary, I encourage you to use your score, whatever it is, to your full advantage. I see it as a jumping-off point, a signal that your skin's brightest days are just ahead.

2

Skin Deep

Just last week, Janine, who is thirty-six years old, walked into my office. Aside from having a few small light-brown spots and faint smile lines, her skin was in great shape for her age. She thought so, too—until she took a good look at her two daughters. Both are under the age of ten, so it'll be years and years before they see their first brown spot or wrinkle. Janine had noticed how much their faces glowed and radiated health, how they lit up every room they walked into—and how, somewhere along the way, her own skin had lost its luster. "Dr. Dover," she said, "I'd give anything to get back even a fraction of that luster."

Most of us can relate to this. If it's not your daughter, maybe it's your niece, your grandchild, or the high schoolers you see walking to class every morning. Think for a minute about a child you know. When you look at his or her face, you probably see the following:

- For starters, you notice an overall radiance. I have two teenage daughters. Like Janine's kids, they have this tremendously healthy luster.

- One of the qualities that makes children look like children is their skin's plumpness. I'm not talking about eating too much cake and ice cream. Youthful skin is filled with goodies like collagen, elastin, and a spongy material called hyaluronic acid, which makes the skin deliciously plump and full. Think of a baby's round cheeks and you'll know just what I mean.

- Plump skin looks healthy and young. It doesn't matter if your daughter has gotten only five hours of sleep or has sunburned her face to a crisp (let's hope not)—her skin is probably still taut and unlined. Of course, all that sun exposure will come back to bite her later on!

- No makeup is necessary to improve one's looks here. One of the most prized aspects of young skin is its lovely even color and tone.

Now let's take a look at how the complexion changes over the decades. The section below outlines how the aging process manifests itself on the skin's surface, as well as below it. If you took my SVA quiz in chapter 1, compare your score with the descriptions below. Do you recognize *your* face?

SVA Breakdown

Twentysomething

Enjoy your skin now; in many ways, it's at its very best. Since it still retains its teenage youthfulness and recoil, makeup is probably not necessary to improve the way it looks. All your face requires to look good is a confident smile. The few creases that appear when you do flash a grin vanish the moment you relax your face. Fortunately, the oil slicks and pimples that were caused mainly by puberty's hormonal shifts have finally begun to abate—for most women, but not all (read on).

Myth   Using a rich moisturizer now will prevent wrinkles later.

Truth   Moisturizers do just what they say they will do: moisturize the skin. Most formulas that contain ingredients like glycerin, petrolatum, and hyaluronic acid hydrate your complexion by helping cells to attract and hold on to water molecules. More moisture in the skin will temporarily make it look more plump, minimizing the appearance of fine lines for up to several hours. Regular use of a moisturizer helps to keep the skin well hydrated over the long term as well. For long-term wrinkle prevention, however, look for a moisturizer that contains anti-aging ingredients, such as retinol and alpha hydroxy acids.

Here are some of the things you'll notice about your skin if your SVA is twentysomething:

- **Persistent pimples.** Acne usually begins to subside at this age, but growing numbers of people are still plagued by blemishes well into their twenties and beyond. Many of my adult patients find that the harsh acne products they depended on in adolescence are too drying and irritating now. Fortunately, we have many gentler alternatives.

- **Sluggish cell turnover.** The natural process of cell turnover begins to slow down very slightly, so dull, dead skin cells stick around for a little longer. This means that your complexion might lose a bit of its natural luster as you approach thirty.

- **Delayed effects of sunburn.** Damage from days spent on the beach starts manifesting itself during this decade. Nevertheless, take heart: any brown spots, fine crinkles, and spidery blood vessels that do emerge are usually barely visible, and further injury is very preventable as long as you get serious about sun protection now.

Thirtysomething

Your complexion still looks youthful: your skin bounces back when you pinch it, and the surface is probably fairly smooth. As you move into your middle and late thirties, however, past sun damage truly begins to make its mark.

If your SVA is thirtysomething, you'll see the following changes in your skin:

- **Luster loss.** Your skin's natural glow and radiance continue to decrease as cell turnover slows down more dramatically.

- **Brown spots.** Although the center of your face is still fairly free of brown spots, the sides show the first signs of pigmentation. The reason for this is that few people ever look directly at the sun, so the sides of the face receive more ultraviolet (UV) exposure. Furthermore, many people neglect the outer part of their cheeks when they apply sunscreen. You'd also be surprised at how much sun exposure happens while you're driving: UVA light transmits right through window glass. Elsewhere on the face, small freckles become larger and more blotchy.

- **Visible veins.** Tiny red veins appear around the edge of the nose and cheeks. At the same time, leg veins might make their first appearance, especially if you've had children.

- **Lines of time.** Fine crinkles start to emerge around the eyes. You might also notice two vertical frown lines between your eyebrows—many of my patients call these their "elevens," because of their shape—and horizontal lines on the forehead that come from raising your eyebrows. All these lines are more noticeable when you're tired, stressed, or dehydrated.

Myth Drinking lots of water will keep me looking young.

Truth Water certainly does the body good, but when it comes to staving off the signs of aging, it's hardly a miracle elixir. Unless you're severely dehydrated—and you'll know it if you are—drinking a little more or a little less than usual really won't show up on your skin. I can't see how drinking eight glasses of water a day would make your skin look younger in the long term. If your complexion is genuinely dry or flaky, the best way to hydrate it is with a good moisturizer, which will help the skin to look smoother and plumper, but only in the short term.

- **Not-so-cute dimples.** Cellulite might appear or become more noticeable, particularly on the back of your thighs and buttocks.

Fortysomething

As years of cumulative UV exposure keep taking their toll, your skin takes on an increasingly dull cast, especially in sun-exposed areas.

If your SVA is fortysomething, you might notice the following happening to your skin:

- **More prevalent pigment.** Brown spots crop up in larger and larger numbers—not only on the sides of your face but also in the central part.
- **Additional wrinkles.** Fine lines continue to emerge, and the overall texture of the skin appears less smooth. Crinkles around the eyes become more noticeable; frown lines between the brows and horizontal creases in the forehead become deeper. You might find it especially frustrating that people are asking you why you look angry when you're perfectly happy.
- **Loss of baby fat.** You might notice gradual volume loss, starting in your cheeks, especially during the later part of the decade. This is when you first start to notice that your skin is visibly less taut, especially around the mouth and along the jawline.

Fiftysomething

The skin is noticeably less radiant than it was a decade ago. Although you might feel as young and vibrant as ever, the hormonal changes associated with menopause, coupled with the ongoing effects of sun exposure from years past, mean that your complexion might look drier and more tired.

Having a fiftysomething SVA often means the following for your skin:

- **Uneven skin tone.** Blotches and redness become even worse as you sail through your fifties. Even if they weren't a problem before, individual red blood vessels can pop up around the nose, cheeks, and chin.

- **More creases.** Forehead lines and crow's feet become deeper, and vertical lip lines might begin to form, especially if they run in your family, if you are or were a smoker, or if you're prone to puckering.
- **Sagging and fat accumulation.** As volume loss continues on the face, neck, and other parts of the body, sagging increases. That's because fat redistributes itself as we age, showing up on different parts of the face and the body. Some of it disappears from the cheeks, causing them to look slightly hollow. At the same time, fat deposits under the eyes and under the chin cause eyelid puffiness and sagging of the neck. Let's also not forget about the areas that are notorious for accumulating fat with age: the belly, the sides of the hips, and the buttocks.

Sixtysomething

The skin looks less radiant and more blotchy than it was a decade ago. Along with these changes comes increased sagging at the corners of the mouth and along the jawline and the neck. All of this is especially disconcerting if you feel as youthful as you did twenty years ago. If you're considering a face-lift or other skin-tightening procedures for the first time, be aware that doctors have a range of less invasive alternatives for those who are not ready to take the cosmetic surgery plunge.

If your SVA is sixtysomething, the following is probably happening to your skin:

- **Deeper lines.** Creases, wrinkles, and frown lines become progressively more etched into your face, especially between the eyebrows, on the forehead, around the eyes and the mouth, and above the upper lip.
- **Unsightly sagging.** Loose skin continues to be more visible on the face, especially along the jawline, on the neck, and throughout the entire body.
- **More fat accumulation.** Even if you're an avid exerciser, you might not be able to stave off emerging "saddlebags" (increased

fat on the sides of the hips) and belly fat as your skin tone decreases and areas of unwanted body fat accumulate.

Seventysomething and Beyond

This decade just brings more of the same. Nevertheless, just because you might be a grandmother doesn't mean that you want to look like one. I still have vivid memories of an older woman who walked into my office and confided that her own grandchildren were too scared to sit on her lap because of the big brown blotches and deep wrinkles on her face.

If your SVA is in the seventies or higher, your skin might exhibit the following:

> **Myth** Topical oxygen treatments will make my skin look younger and healthier.
>
> **Truth** Our cells, including our skin cells, obviously can't function without oxygen, but they get plenty of it from our bloodstream. There's no evidence that rubbing or spraying your face with oxygen does a thing, which is why I refuse to let our office aestheticians offer any type of oxygenating treatments.

- **Unstoppable spots.** Uneven pigmentation usually becomes more noticeable as you move through your seventies, with darker, raised, and even blotchier spots.

- **Red veins.** Facial vessels appear or become more noticeable around the nose and on the cheeks, even if they weren't a problem before.

- **More wrinkles.** Sensing a pattern here? Creases are prominent on the brow, on the forehead, between the nose and the mouth, on the cheeks, and especially above the upper lip. For those who have expressive faces or who have had lots of sun exposure over the years, the face becomes more and more wrinkly. Alas, the makeup you once wore to cover the brown spots and to mask small imperfections now accentuates them.

- **Sagging skin.** The areas around the brows, cheeks, jawline, and neck continue to droop even more.

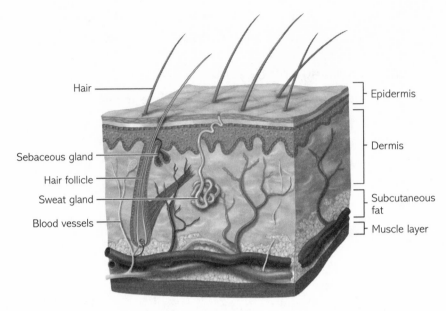

Hair

Epidermis

Dermis

Sebaceous gland

Hair follicle

Sweat gland

Blood vessels

Subcutaneous fat

Muscle layer

A cross-section model of the layers of the skin.

How Your Skin Functions as You Age

I'm not telling you all of this to make you pine for your younger days. However, before we figure out your personalized equation for lowering your SVA, it helps to know how *all* skin functions during childhood and adolescence, when skin is at its peak, and how skin changes as it ages. First, we need a quick biology lesson; bear with me on this. The skin is made up of three layers: the epidermis, the dermis, and subcutaneous fat.

The outermost layer is the epidermis, whose function is mainly to keep harmful material from entering your body. The epidermis is mostly made up of cells called keratinocytes, which shed and regenerate regularly. Cells turn over most rapidly in younger skin. Although you can't actually see dead cells shedding on a day-to-day basis, you know it's happening because of the telltale luminous glow that results from having new cells. As the process of cell turnover gradually slows down during your twenties, thirties, and beyond, the complexion can begin to look duller.

When Bad Things Happen to Good Cells

Kristin, an Irish American, had beautiful, fair skin. During the past several years, she had become meticulous about applying sunscreen every day. At the beach, she always wore a big floppy straw hat and sat under an umbrella. In short, Kristin was a model patient. Nothing, however, could change the fact that Kristin was a reformed sun addict, so she wasn't entirely shocked the day she was in my office for one of her routine mole checks and we found a suspicious spot that turned out to be skin cancer. We were just thankful that we caught it early.

A well-functioning epidermis keeps harmful viruses, bacteria, and foreign and unwanted substances from attacking the rest of the body. Sometimes, however, our well-meaning epidermal cells turn on us and begin mutating, or reproducing improperly; this is almost always caused by excessive sun exposure, which sets the stage for abnormal cellular growths that occasionally turn into skin cancer.

Mutations in keratinocytes account for the two most common forms of the disease: basal cell and squamous cell carcinoma. More than a million Americans develop these two types of skin cancer every year. Most of these skin tumors are easily treatable when they are found early. Resistant or untreated growths can invade other parts of the body or leave unsightly scars behind.

Melanoma, the third most common—and the most dangerous—form of skin cancer, develops when melanocytes take a wrong turn and begin to mutate. It's almost 100 percent curable when it's diagnosed early, but when it spreads to other parts of the body, the disease can be fatal. About sixty thousand Americans are diagnosed every year with melanoma, resulting in more than eight thousand deaths.

The good news is that skin cancer is not only treatable, it's preventable. UV light exposure is responsible for almost all basal cell and squamous cell carcinomas and at least a significant number of melanomas, which appear most often on the face, ears, neck, scalp, shoulders, and back. This makes protective clothing and sunscreen required gear whenever you work or play outside, even if it's a cloudy day. An added bonus is that you're not only preventing skin cancer, you're keeping your SVA beautifully low. See pages 110–111 for more on how to distinguish a garden-variety mole or scaly patch from skin cancer.

Myth   Facial exercises will keep my complexion from sagging.

Truth   If regular trips to the gym keep your abdominal muscles, biceps, and thighs firm and toned, you'd think that exercising the muscles of the face would operate on the same principle. Unfortunately, it's not that easy. The main culprit behind facial sagging is not loss of muscle tone but loss of collagen, elastin, and fat, and much of this is due to genetics and (to a lesser extent) sun exposure. Certain topical ingredients, like DMAE and GABA, which are found in skin-tightening cosmeceuticals, will help to make your complexion more taut, at least temporarily. Now there are also in-office skin-tightening procedures, such as Thermage, Titan, and ReFirme, that can significantly tighten hanging skin in one appointment or over the course of a few appointments, depending on the device used.

Sprinkled among all those keratinocytes are melanocytes, which are responsible for your skin color, are a handful of Langerhans cells, which regulate immune responses in the skin.

The dermis, the layer just below the epidermis, is made up of collagen, elastin fibers, and blood vessels. Collagen and elastin sit in a thick gel called hyaluronic acid. Together they make your skin spongy and plump. Like your epidermis, your dermis is also constantly turning over, replenishing blood vessels, collagen, and elastic fibers. However, with age—and especially with exposure to sun, cigarette smoke, and other environmental assaults—the turnover process slows down. Some blood vessels might shrink and disappear; the remaining ones will dilate, making mature complexions more prone to red blotches. Fewer well-functioning blood vessels means that your skin takes longer to heal and respond to sun damage, which is part of the reason your collagen and elastin gradually accumulate injury with age. Meanwhile, the cushiony hyaluronic acid diminishes, making the skin less spongy. This explains why aging skin not only develops increasing numbers of fine lines but also becomes saggy and crepelike just beneath the surface.

The third layer of the skin, subcutaneous fat, sits underneath the dermis and varies in amount, depending on your physique and the location of the skin on your body. Although this layer might be the least loved component of our skin, subcutaneous fat holds our larger blood vessels and nerves, and it also serves the critical purpose of absorbing shocks and insulating the body from cold. Depending on how this fat is housed inside its pockets of connective tissue, it can begin to pucker and dimple, resulting in cellulite, which is notoriously difficult to eliminate. As many of my female patients know, cellulite can make an appearance even if you're relatively lean and fit. Worst of all is that the condition tends to amplify with age.

In part, your genes determine whether your skin's virtual age will rise right along with your actual age. Heredity has a lot to do with when lines, brown spots, sagging, and cellulite emerge—if at all. Therefore, if your mom could pass for your older sister, consider yourself lucky. Avoiding cigarette smoke and excessive exposure to the sun will slow down the aging process considerably, keeping your SVA low.

There are also countless proactive measures you can take to prevent and even reverse the passage of time. Many patients, for example, are now having a man-made version of the body's own hyaluronic acid injected directly into fine lines, wrinkles, and the lips to replenish what Mother Nature has taken away. For those who aren't ready to face the syringe, topical products—like moisturizers spiked with hyaluronic acid to hydrate and temporarily plump the skin a bit—can

Puckering

Puckering can hasten the development of fine vertical lines above the upper lip. Smoking is one of the biggest culprits: not only does it require frequent pursing of the lips, but the smoke itself breaks down collagen and elastin fibers. In addition, female smokers tend to go through menopause earlier than other women, which is another cause of premature aging. Drinking from a straw also brings on those upper-lip lines. In fact, most of us pucker our lips when we speak without even knowing it. Botox injections in the upper lip help to limit puckering, while preserving other natural movements of the lips. Over time the injections will actually decrease these lines. It might sound excessive, but it really works.

make a world of difference. When my patient Janine asked me whether it was possible to reclaim her complexion's lost luster, I sent her home with a simple regimen: a mild cleanser for the morning and evening, a sunscreen with anti-aging ingredients, and a retinoid to use at bedtime. A week later, she was already noticing tiny improvements. I can't wait to see her in another six weeks.

I applied the same philosophy to Janine's skin that I do to all of my patients: if you're proactive today about nurturing your complexion, tomorrow will look a whole lot brighter. That means adopting a ridiculously simple, but marvelously effective, basic skin-care regimen. Once you have this regimen in place, you can continue to adjust it to suit the changing needs of your complexion, but the fundamental steps should always remain in place. I think of it as a tripod with very sturdy legs.

The three activities of a basic skin-care regimen are the following:

1. **Cleanse.** Cleansers are not all created equal. Find the right formula for your face and learn how to maximize its effectiveness.

2. **Treat.** You should have a morning and a night treatment program. The latest lotions, creams, and serums repair and rejuvenate the skin, giving new meaning to the term *beauty sleep*. No twelve-hour period should pass without your applying an effective skin treatment that helps to reverse and prevent skin damage and aging.

3. **Prevent**. Sunscreen is the single most important anti-aging weapon you can buy. With so many light and nongreasy versions available now, there's no excuse *not* to wear it every day.

This is simple, right? The only tricky part, really, is choosing the right products and, most important, making them as much a part of your routine as brushing your teeth every morning and night. This is why I have devoted a comprehensive chapter to each crucial step. As your skin changes, you will probably have to reassess your treatment regimen. The cleanser you use at age twenty-five will not necessarily suit you in your forties. Thus, I encourage you to revisit chapter 3,

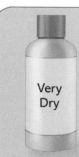

For the driest, most sensitive types, the cleansers with the kindest touch are the surfactant-free, tissue-off formulas (no rinsing required). These rich washes not only preserve your skin's moisture but may also add extra hydration by building up your protective lipid barrier.

Very Dry

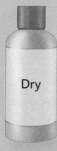

If your skin is easily irritated and a bit dry, choose a creamy wash. Many are surfactant free, so they won't aggravate sensitive or rosacea-plagued skin. They rinse away without washing all of your natural fatty oils down the drain. Rest assured: While your face may not feel "squeaky clean" after using them, these formulas still do an excellent job of removing dirt and debris.

Dry

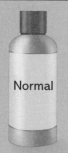

Normal-to-oily skin is a perfect candidate for foaming cleansers that effectively lift away surface grime. And if your skin also happens to be sensitive, look for some the newest formulas made without surfactants.

Normal

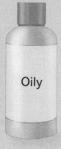

Oily or pimple-prone skin? Choose a clear, noncreamy cleanser. Many come spiked with anti-acne ingredients like salicylic acid or benzoyl peroxide, which break down sebum and other pore-cloggin muck.

Oily

The cleanser spectrum, from very dry to oily.

"Cleanse," whenever you think that your needs have changed: when your skin begins to look dry, irritated, broken out, or just plain dull. What good is a basic treatment regimen if it doesn't support your complexion properly as your skin changes?

The Dermatologist

Janine's story at the beginning of this chapter is not only inspiring, it also proves just how much of a difference finding the right skin-care regimen can make. This book gives you the tools for designing your own SVA-lowering plan without a doctor's help. After all, if you're basically happy with your skin, there's no need to see a dermatologist. Nevertheless, there might be times when you want to book an appointment, such as to get a prescription for the type of topical retinoid cream I gave to Janine or to address another issue.

Dermatologists are undoubtedly the world's foremost experts in the treatment of skin, hair, and nails. A dermatologist is therefore the first person to call if you have a problem with any of those areas. That means booking appointments for regular skin cancer screenings or to

Myth   The more facials I get, the younger my skin will look.

Truth   That might be true short-term. Done properly, a good facial can cleanse and brighten the skin temporarily, as well as reduce stress. It's a safe bet that you'll leave the spa looking like a refreshed, more youthful version of yourself. Just don't expect that pampering treatment to keep fine lines from emerging. Also, be aware that some facials can actually cause breakouts, irritation, or even permanent scarring. My advice is to avoid treatments that involve pore extractions—and if you leave the spa looking worse than you did when you walked in, don't go back. Alternatives to facials are glycolic acid peels, microdermabrasion, and vibraderm treatments, which, when done properly and fairly aggressively, alter the structure of the skin. All these treatments can make a slight but significant improvement in the skin, both short-term and long-term.

check out a new rash, spot, growth, or bump. (Anyone with a personal or family history of skin cancer should have a body check at least once a year.) You can also consult a dermatologist for all kinds of skin problems, such as acne and rosacea, hair and scalp problems, such as hair thinning, or if you suspect you're developing a nail fungus. But as the field of cosmetic dermatology advances, we're increasingly called upon to address issues that are not strictly medical, such as skin discoloration and skin aging. These days, dermatologists are more educated and better equipped than ever when it comes to softening, and even erasing, the signs of aging. That can mean focusing on preventative steps to help you age more slowly and gracefully so that you can postpone or eliminate the need for more aggressive procedures in the future.

Type *dermatologist* and your zip code into any online search engine, and you'll be given a long list of doctors' names, addresses, and phone numbers—and very little else. Here's how to start separating the true skin gurus from the rest of the pack:

- **Check for certification**. Check with the American Academy of Dermatology (www.aad.org) and the American Society for Dermatologic Surgery (www.asds.net). Both groups keep lists of board-certified dermatologists and dermatologic surgeons.

- **Ask around.** The best medical pedigree doesn't mean anything if your doctor has no bedside manner or isn't up on the latest skin science. Call trusted friends (the ones with great complexions, of course), family members, and your primary care doctor to see which dermatologists they recommend.

- **Go online.** These days, most physicians have incredibly informative Web sites that tell you everything from where they went to school to what books they're writing. These sites not only reveal information about your potential dermatologist's skill but also might give you a peek at his or her personality. Just remember not to take *everything* you read on the Internet at face value. Some so-called independent sites that claim to review doctors might simply have an ax to grind.

- **Consider location.** People have certainly traveled from other countries to get my advice, but in general I suggest finding a doctor in your area. Otherwise, a quick lunchtime appointment can turn into an all-day affair.
- **Know when to cut your losses.** If you find the dermatologist of your dreams, only to later discover that he or she is not for you, don't be afraid to look some more. You should feel absolutely comfortable with your doctor; if you don't, switch. After all, it's your body, your skin, your face—and your money.

Here's a story about a patient who wound up in my office: A well-dressed thirtysomething patient named Suzanne came to see me not long ago. I'm exaggerating only slightly when I say that she toted a suitcase on wheels and a magnifying mirror the size of a flat-screen television. I don't know how she lifted the things out of her car. When I looked at her quizzically, she said, "Unless I use this mirror, I won't be able to show you what bothers me." Think about that for a minute. Suzanne needed a mirror that magnifies every "flaw"—every pore, blemish, and wrinkle—to *ten times* its actual size just to show me where her trouble spots were. If you ask me, what she really needed was counseling.

The vast majority of people who come to see me, however, have fairly routine and rational concerns. Sometimes the hardest part of my work is making sure that all their concerns are addressed during their limited time in the examination room. My advice to you as a patient, therefore, is to be realistic about the amount of time you'll have with your dermatologist. Expecting a consultation to last an hour and a half is not realistic. Even half an hour is a bit too optimistic. A more reasonable time frame is fifteen minutes, which is generally plenty of time to explain your goals, have your skin assessed, and walk out with the information you need.

Although a really good doctor will ask you what bothers you most about your skin, it's a good idea to consider in advance precisely how you'd like to go about lowering your SVA. Think about what your specific goals are. Even if you can think of many, resist the temptation to bring in a long list—otherwise, your doctor won't be able to devote a significant amount of time to any one concern. Instead, choose a few specific things that bother you most. It might help to write them down on a small index card. As you get to know the doctor and his or her staff, and after your most important items have been addressed, you can start to focus on some of the other issues that are on your mind.

Keep in mind that the more precise you are when you outline your goals, the happier you'll be—and the sooner you'll start to see your SVA plummet. Here's one example: Not long ago, a forty-year-old patient named Evelyn was sitting in my chair for her first Botox injection. Minutes before I was about to begin, she looked me in the eye and said, "I want to tell you something really important. You know this 'looking natural' thing? Forget it. I don't care about looking natural. I want to look perfect. I hate these lines." She wasn't joking, either. She was completely serious. This was one of the most surprising things a patient has ever

Myth   Sunglasses are the key to keeping future crow's feet at bay.

Truth   This one has at least some truth to it. Besides helping to prevent cataracts, a good pair of shades with UVA and UVB protection will reduce your need to squint, which might slow the formation of crow's feet, and will shield the area immediately around the eyes from sun damage. However, you'd need a pretty big pair of Jackie O–type sunglasses to make a significant difference. It's much easier—and more effective—to zap those fine lines with Botox.

told me. One hundred people will tell me not to overdo it with the Botox or any other treatments we are planning to do—and that is exactly my philosophy—but then the next person will make the exact opposite request. When I'm removing a patient's brown spots, she might tell me to start by taking off just a few because she's scared to see herself without all the freckles she's used to—or she might ask me to erase all of them. The bottom line: ask for what you want.

Finally, pay close attention to the advice your dermatologist gives you. Every once in a while a patient will want to tape-record our conversation, or she'll scribble so furiously as I speak that I'm positive she

Myth I can keep my skin looking young by changing my sleep position.

Truth This one sounds weird, but it's true. "Sleep wrinkles" or "sleep creases" actually exist, and they form when your face is squished into the same position, night after night, for years. A predominant crease that runs down and across the forehead and one that runs from the cheek to the lip are two examples of sleep-induced creases. You can prevent them by sleeping on your other side or on your back, resting your head on a satin or silk pillowcase. A very soft fabric, such as satin or silk, will not crease your facial skin when you sleep on the side of your face. Sleep creases are caused by the face being crunched by a pillow, and over time they leave permanent, deep facial lines. If you want more immediate improvement, you can have the creases filled with one of several filler substances (see pages 183–189 for more information).

can't possibly be processing a word I say. Personally, I think you'll get much more out of the appointment if you sit back and just listen. If you're truly worried that you'll forget everything by the time you get home, tell your doctor. After I finish talking with a patient, I'm always happy to write down my instructions or send him or her a typed letter that sums up the appointment and the treatment plan.

The Game Plan: Six Do-at-Home Steps for Lowering Your SVA

1. ID your SVA. Before you even start to save your skin, you have to really know your SVA. If you haven't done so already, take my quiz in chapter 1 to get your score, then read my descriptions of the issues that typically crop up during *your* decade—and why.

2. Stop smoking. Not only does exposure to cigarette smoke break down the collagen and elastin fibers that make your skin malleable, the constant puckering of the lips to hold the cigarette in your mouth hastens the formation of upper-lip lines.

3. Embrace my philosophy: cleanse, treat, prevent. Even my least disciplined patients can manage to do this extremely simple, yet enormously effective, three-step plan: cleanse, treat, prevent. It's a mantra you'll see me repeat over and over, because it works.

4. Pick the right doctor. Although you can follow this program on your own, finding a dermatologist with the right credentials, knowledge, skill set, bedside manner, and ingenuity will go a very long way toward lowering your skin's virtual age quickly and dramatically.

5. Choose your "big three." If you try hard enough, I'm sure you could come up with many skin issues you'd like to fix. However, if you really want to make a difference in your complexion, choose the three things that bother you the most so that you and your dermatologist can devise a focused plan. Most important, don't get caught up in useless and sometimes pricey gimmicks that promise to make you look younger. Guzzling ten glasses of imported spring water every day won't turn back the clock, nor will the fanciest facial. Diligently using the right products will.

6. Pay attention. As obvious as it sounds, once you find a dermatologist you trust, listen to him or her. If you don't understand the instructions you receive, clarify them before you leave or even after the appointment is over. After all, even the best anti-aging plan won't work if you can't remember it or if it's too complicated to follow.

3

Cleanse

In one hand, you have an ordinary bar of soap. In the other, you have a creamy face wash. Both lather well; both lift away dirt and oil. However, the two will most definitely not affect your complexion in the same way. The right cleanser for you depends on how your skin is behaving now: whether it's oily, dry, or somewhere in between; whether it's sensitive or hardy; whether the time of year is summer or winter; and whether your SVA is significantly lower than, higher than, or equivalent to your actual age.

Before we go any further, it's time to discover how much you really know about skin cleansers and what they can and can't do to make you look younger. So sharpen your pencil and take this quick quiz. Do not skip ahead to look at the answers!

1. Washing my face twice a day can do what for my SVA?

A. Lower it dramatically

B. Diminish it slightly

C. Nothing—but I will have cleaner, fresher-looking skin

2. Which type of cleanser ingredients helps to turn back the clock?

   A. Moisturizers

   B. Exfoliants like alpha hydroxy acids

   C. Anti-acne ingredients like salicylic acid or benzoyl peroxide, along with all of the above

3. If I'm going to skip my cleansing step once a day, which is the better time to skip?

   A. The evening

   B. The morning

   C. I can actually skip both morning and evening if my skin is normal and behaving well

4. After washing my face, my skin should feel

   A. Extremely tight

   B. Slightly tight

   C. As if I just applied a light coat of moisturizing cream

5. A surfactant is

   A. A detergent that breaks down and washes away my skin's natural oils

   B. A grainy scrub that sloughs away dead skin cells

   C. The residue left in the sink after I wash my face

6. Most skin types can handle a gentle exfoliating scrub at least

   A. Twice per day

   B. Two or three times per week

   C. Only once per month

7. The advantage of using an exfoliating cleanser is that it

   A. Completely erases wrinkles over time

   B. Can "scrub away" a severe case of acne

   C. Helps a dull complexion to become more radiant and dewy

8. Which of these tasks can a cleanser not accomplish?

   A. Fade visible sun damage with exfoliants

B. Help to prevent sun damage with antioxidants

C. Block UV light with sunblock

9. Blended into cleansers, fruit extracts like papaya and pineapple

   A. Contain enzymes that help to unglue dead skin cells and other debris

   B. Make cleansers less appealing to use

   C. Are just a sweet-smelling gimmick and offer no real benefit

10. What is the main difference between physical and chemical exfoliating cleansers?

    A. Chemical exfoliants should be used only under the supervision of a dermatologist.

    B. The former contains beads or grains, whereas the latter has safe levels of gentle acids.

    C. There is no difference.

Answers

1. B: Cleansers aren't miracle workers. Since much of the formula washes down the drain, it won't smooth away fine lines as dramatically as the right treatment lotion, serum, or cream will do. Some cleansers do leave small amounts of active ingredients behind on the face. Even if you use a mild cleanser without treatment benefits, whisking away the dirt and oil on your face will help any lotions or creams you apply afterward to be absorbed into the skin and work more efficiently.

2. B: Moisturizers can make wrinkles less apparent for a few hours, and anti-acne ingredients will help to clear your skin, but only exfoliants will help your skin to look younger long-term by evening out discoloration and gradually improving texture.

3. B: I encourage all my patients, except those with extremely dry skin, to cleanse morning and night. If you must skip one, make it the morning wash. It's imperative that you take the time every night to remove makeup, excess oil, and the environmental debris that has accumulated on your face throughout the day.

4. B: Aim for a pleasantly tight feeling after cleansing. If your face stings or feels uncomfortably taut, your cleanser is too drying. If you look shiny minutes after washing, your formula is too rich for your skin type.

5. A: The word *detergent* might sound harsh, but cleansers come in a wide range of surfactant levels, from very low to high.

6. B: Although sensitive skin types might be able to handle only occasional exfoliating—or sometimes none at all—most complexions do well with a gentle exfoliant two or three times per week.

7. C: Exfoliating cleansers can't erase wrinkles. If used too aggressively, they can irritate the skin, causing redness and swelling, and aggravate existing pimples. Used properly—as long as your skin isn't too sensitive—these scrubs can certainly restore a youthful glow to dull, aging skin.

8. C: Unfortunately, we haven't yet found a way to formulate a cleanser that leaves sunblock behind on the skin. However, washes that contain antioxidants can help to prevent sun damage. A good exfoliating cleanser can help to fade sun spots and fine lines for a long time.

9. A: Cleansers that contain fruit extracts *do* smell good, which makes washing your face feel like a pampering treat. Nevertheless, that's not where the benefits end. These ingredients have powerful enzymes that help exfoliate dead skin cells and dirt, making any treatment product you apply afterward work much more effectively.

10. B: Cleansers that contain smooth beads or grains are physical exfoliants, whereas those with gentle acids or enzymes are chemical exfoliants. Both methods work well. Continue reading to determine which might be best for your skin type.

Why Cleanse?

I vividly remember the day that Lydia walked into my office. A high-powered and high-profile CEO, this fortysomething patient desperately wanted to know how she could spruce up her appearance, especially because younger, junior-level employees were quickly making their way up the corporate ladder. Lydia had the money and the drive to undergo any fancy anti-aging procedure I could dish out: Botox, lasers, you name it. You can imagine my shock when I casually asked what type of cleanser she washed her face with, and she sheepishly admitted that she lathered up with whatever bar of soap she had in the shower in the morning and never bothered to wash her face before bed. "Who has time?" she asked me, shrugging her shoulders. "Besides, compared to all the high-tech creams and treatments out there, what difference will washing the face even make?"

I'm astounded by the number of patients who say nearly the same thing. They look me in the eye and admit that they routinely collapse into bed after a late night without so much as cracking open a face wash. These are otherwise bright people who invest a great deal of energy in their physical appearance. They make time for manicures, hair color appointments, and gym workouts. Yet they slack off when it comes to the simplest, easiest kind of skin maintenance. Unless they break out in pimples from all the dirt and makeup they leave caked inside their pores, cleansing sometimes becomes an afterthought. Little do they know that this simple step is one of the easiest, no-brainer ways to lower their skin's virtual age.

Washing your face twice daily is ideal, but the most important time to care for your skin is at night, particularly if you plan on significantly decreasing your SVA. Think about it: Your face has probably spent the day coated in some kind of makeup, moisturizing cream, and, I hope, sunscreen. Smog and other environmental pollutants have settled onto your skin's surface. You've most likely touched your face several times throughout the day, leaving behind a layer of oil and bacteria.

Now imagine falling into bed and pressing your cheek against your pillowcase, embedding all kinds of gunk into your defenseless pores. It's a miracle if your complexion doesn't wind up duller over time.

Furthermore, by whisking away the day's dirt and debris, properly cleansing the face before going to bed ensures that any treatment product you put on afterward will be easily absorbed into the skin so that it can go right to work on any trouble spots. The period you spend in bed every night represents eight hours, give or take, of uninterrupted skin repair time. This repair time can mean the difference between seeing your first wrinkle at age twenty-eight or thirty-eight. It can leave the most mature skin looking radiant and sparkling. I challenge any face-washing slackers to start sudsing up twice a day for six weeks, then retake my SVA quiz. You *will* see a difference in your score—as long as you choose the right cleanser, that is.

I remember a forty-three-year-old patient named Mary Ellen, who had spent the past decade of her life washing her face with a bar of Dial soap. Deodorant soap might be acceptable from the neck down (although I prefer moisturizing body washes), but it can be murder on the face. Her skin had become so parched that her emerging fine lines were especially noticeable. In addition, her cheeks looked red and flaky. The first thing I did was send her home with a rich cream cleanser. That alone made her skin look creamier in just one week, lowering her SVA by a year or two. The effects were not dramatic, but they were not bad, considering that all she did was give up the bar of harsh deodorant soap.

Cleansers have come a long way in the past few years. There are a variety of gentle bar soaps specifically designed for the face, and the liquid washes also come in many wonderful varieties (such as foamy, granular, creamy, lotions or clear). Some fight pimples, soothe sensitive skin, or claim to smooth away fine lines. There are even some multi-tasking formulas that promise a combination of all these things. Although there's a cleanser to fit every skin type, the sheer number of them is overwhelming enough to make some people resort to the bar soap they use on the rest of their body, like Mary Ellen's yellow hunk of Dial.

This doesn't mean that strong cleansers are totally bad for your face. Nearly all contain some amount of surfactant, or detergent, which breaks down and washes away your skin's natural oils—and with them, dirt and debris. The more surfactants a cleanser has, the better it works. Yet if you are sensitive to these cleaning ingredients, a high-surfactant formula might irritate your skin, making it blotchy and flaky.

How do you know whether a cleanser is doing more harm than good? After rinsing it away, watch the clock. If your face feels pleasantly tight for ten to fifteen minutes, you've successfully removed much of its surface oil and dirt. If the tightness feels unpleasant or itchy, or if it lasts longer than fifteen minutes, consult the list of cleansers in "Dr. Dover Recommends" that follows to find something gentler. If you feel no tightness at all, and you're constantly battling acne and shine, consider looking for a formula with a bit more strength.

For the driest, most sensitive types of skin, the cleansers with the kindest touch are the surfactant-free, tissue-off formulas, no rinsing required. These rich washes not only preserve your skin's moisture but also add extra hydration by building up your protective lipid barrier.

If your skin is easily irritated and a bit dry, choose a creamy wash. Many are surfactant-free, so they won't aggravate sensitive or rosacea-plagued skin. They rinse away without washing all of your natural fatty oils down the drain. Be assured that even though your face might not feel "squeaky clean" after using them, these formulas still do an excellent job of removing dirt and debris.

Normal to oily skin is a perfect candidate for foaming cleansers that effectively lift away surface grime. If your skin also happens to be sensitive, look for some of the newest formulas made without surfactants.

If you have oily or pimple-prone skin, choose a clear, noncreamy cleanser. Many come spiked with anti-acne ingredients like salicylic acid or benzoyl peroxide, which break down sebum and other pore-clogging muck.

Dr. Dover Recommends

Drugstore

Normal Skin
- Skin Effects Gentle Foaming Cleanser for Normal Skin
- Skin Effects Deep-Cleaning Enzyme Scrub
- Skin Effects Self-Heating Resurfacing Cleanser
- Olay Daily Facials Express Wet Cleansing Cloths for All Skin Types
- Olay Regenerist Daily Regenerating Cleanser
- Olay Regenerist Night Recovery Moisturizing Treatment
- Cetaphil Daily Facial Cleanser for Normal to Oily Skin
- Pond's Clean Sweep, Cleansing & Make-Up Removing Towelettes

Oily Skin
- Olay Daily Facials Deep Cleansing Cloths for Combination/Oily Skin
- La Roche-Posay Effaclar Purifying Foaming Gel

Dry Skin
- Skin Effects Deep-Cleaning Enzyme Scrub
- Eucerin Gentle Hydrating Cleanser
- Neutrogena One Step Gentle Cleanser

Combination Skin
- Skin Effects Deep-Cleaning Enzyme Scrub
- Skin Effects Gentle Foaming Cleanser
- L'Oreal Ideal Balance Foaming Cream Cleanser

Sensitive Skin
- Skin Effects Redness Control Calming Gel Cleanser
- Olay Foaming Face Wash for Sensitive Skin
- Neutrogena Extra Gentle Cleanser, Fragrance Free
- Cetaphil Gentle Skin Cleanser
- Vichy Calming Cleansing Solution

Acne-Prone Skin
- Skin Effects Acne Cleansing Daily Mask
- L'Oreal Pure Zone Unclogging Scrub Cleanser
- Neutrogena Rapid Clear Oil-Control Foaming Cleanser
- Aveeno Active Naturals Clear Complexion Foaming Cleanser
- Olay Total Effects Anti-Aging Anti-Blemish Daily Cleanser
- La Roche-Posay Biomedic Antibac Acne Wash

Bar Soaps
- Dove Beauty Bar
- La Roche-Posay Lipikar Surgras Cleansing Bar
- Purpose Gentle Cleansing Bar
- Olay Body Ultra Moisture Moisturizing Bar with Shea Butter

Body Washes
- Aveeno Active Naturals Skin Relief Body Wash
- Olay Moisturinse in Shower Body Lotion with Shea Butter
- Olay Body Quench Body Wash
- Aveeno Active Naturals Eczema Care Body Wash

Department Store and Doctor's Office

Normal Skin
- SkinCare Prescription System Cleanser
- SkinMedica Facial Cleanser
- SkinCeuticals Foaming Cleanser

Oily Skin
- DDF Blemish Foaming Cleanser
- La Mer The Cleansing Fluid
- RéVive Cleanser Agressif

Dry Skin
- Patricia Wexler M.D. Dermatology Universal Anti-Aging Cleanser

- N.V. Perricone M.D. Olive Oil Polyphenols Gentle Cleanser
- La Prairie Cellular Comforting Cleansing Emulsion
- Clé de Peau Gentle Cleansing Foam
- RéVive Cleanser Crème Luxe

Combination Skin
- SkinCeuticals Simply Clean
- La Mer The Cleansing Foam

Sensitive Skin
- SkinMedica Sensitive Skin Cleanser
- Dr. Brandt Lineless Gel Cleanser
- SkinCeuticals Gentle Cleanser
- N.V. Perricone M.D. Vitamin C Ester Citrus Facial Wash
- La Prairie Cellular Cleansing Water for Eyes & Face
- La Mer The Cleansing Lotion

Acne-Prone Skin
- SkinMedica Acne Foaming Wash
- SkinCeuticals Clarifying Cleanser
- Murad Clarifying Cleanser
- Patricia Wexler M.D. Dermatology Acnescription Exfoliating Acne Cleanser

Bar Soaps
- Sisley Botanical Soapless Facial Cleansing Bar

Body Washes
- Murad Acne Body Wash

Exfoliants

There's another element to think about when you're choosing your cleanser: exfoliation. The way that skin-care companies toss around this word, you'd think it was some kind of magic trick that will make your grandmother's face look like a teenager's. Exfoliation won't work miracles, but it can definitely help to brighten your skin. An exfoliant is basically anything that helps to take off the uppermost layers of skin, thus speeding up cell turnover, which begins to slow down during your twenties. An exfoliant can make a complexion that has begun to look duller with age look more radiant, bright, and dewy. I liken these over-the-counter scrubs to a good polish for your finest set of silver. An exfoliant won't erase wrinkles or lines on the surface, but used delicately, it keeps "tarnish" at bay and can even knock a year or two off of your SVA.

Let's run through the three types of exfoliants: physical, chemical, and enzyme.

Physical Exfoliants

Unlike some old-school physical exfoliants, whose jagged seeds and grains caused hundreds of tiny cuts in the skin, the newer versions use soft, perfectly spherical beads to gently abrade top dead skin cells without irritating the skin.

Physical exfoliants are best for thicker skin types that don't abrade easily, skin that is not easily irritated, acne-prone and oily skin, and skin that is sensitive to chemical and enzyme exfoliants. Even women with the most sensitive skin can usually use these types of gentle cleansers without irritation.

Watch out if you have thin, fine, or extremely sensitive skin. Physical exfoliants are okay to use if you have active pimples, but be careful, because they might rupture if you scrub too vigorously.

Chemical Exfoliants

Chemical exfoliants contain low concentrations of alpha and beta hydroxy acids, like glycolic, salicylic, or citric acid, or a combination. The acids help to gently exfoliate the upper layers of the skin.

Chemical exfoliants are best for those whose skin can't tolerate abrasive beads or those who are prone to acne. Salicylic acid, which dissolves the sticky oils inside pores, can be especially helpful in controlling pimples.

Watch out if you are easily irritated by these ingredients, have rosacea, or flush easily (see pages 86–87 for more information about rosacea).

Enzyme Exfoliants

Enzyme exfoliants contain enzymes from pineapple, papaya, and pumpkin as well as other botanical extracts. These enzymes loosen dead skin cells and other debris. Unless you happen to be allergic to one of the extracts, they also tend to be quite gentle, and they usually smell wonderful.

Enzyme exfoliants are best for those who want gentle cleansing and a nice fragrant treat at the same time.

Watch out if you are sensitive to the active ingredient itself. Otherwise, you should tolerate one of these cleansers very well.

How and When to Exfoliate

No matter which type you choose, you shouldn't necessarily use an exfoliating cleanser twice a day, every day of the week. Overscrubbing will make your complexion red and blotchy at best. At worst, it will leave you raw and prone to allergic sensitization, or even infection. In these cases, exfoliation can actually *increase* your SVA, just as Mary Ellen's deodorant soap did. When my patients ask how much is too much, I tell them to watch their skin. Sensitive types might want to stick with their gentle, nonabrading wash, then try a gentle scrub once a week—perhaps on the weekend when they have time to pamper themselves. (If you're using that scrub on sensitive skin for the first time, it might even be a good idea to use the scrub on a Saturday, two days before returning to work on Monday, in case the cleanser leaves the skin looking a little red and flaky.) In fact, for any skin type, I often suggest keeping two different cleansers on hand: a milder one, designed to gently wash away excess oil and debris, and a stronger one, geared toward improving the overall integrity of the skin.

Scrub morning or night, whichever you prefer. Some of my patients like to perform a facial scrub and sometimes a body scrub in the morning; a tingly one helps them to wake up. One benefit to doing it at night, however, is that it paves the way for any night treatment product that you apply immediately afterward to penetrate and work more efficiently while you sleep.

Dr. Dover Recommends

Drugstore

Physical Exfoliants
- Skin Effects Resurfacing Effects Skin Renewal System
- Olay Smooth Skin Exfoliating Scrub with Gentle Microbeads
- Olay Definity Pore Redefining Scrub
- Aveeno Skin Brightening Daily Scrub
- RoC Daily Microdermabrasion Cleansing Disks
- La Roche-Posay Biomedic Micro Exfoliating Scrub

Chemical Exfoliants
- Neutrogena Healthy Skin Visibly Even Foaming Cleanser
- La Roche-Posay Biomedic LHA Cleansing Gel
- Pond's Dramatic Results Age-Defying Cleansing Towelettes with Vitamin A, Retinol, and Collagen

Enzyme Exfoliants
- Skin Effects Deep-Cleaning Enzyme Scrub
- RoC Age Diminishing Facial Cleanser
- Neutrogena Healthy Skin Visibly Even Skin Polishing Enzyme Treatment

Department Store and Doctor's Office

Physical Exfoliants
- SkinCare Prescription System Exfoliator
- SkinMedica Skin Polisher
- Dr. Brandt Microdermabrasion
- Clé de Peau Refreshing Cleansing Foam
- Sisley Botanical Buff & Wash Facial Gel
- RéVive Cleanser Exfoliante

Chemical Exfoliants
- SkinCeuticals Cleansing Cream

- DDF Glycolic 5% Daily Cleansing Pads
- N.V. Perricone M.D. Pore Refining Cleanser
- Patricia Wexler M.D. Dermatology Dual Action Foaming Cleanser

Decoding Ingredient Lists

Take out your favorite skin-care product box and try to read the entire ingredient list aloud—not fun, right? I've been a dermatologist for more than twenty years, and even I can think of hundreds of things I'd rather do than sound out terms like *pentaerythrityl tetrastearate*.

This does not mean that you should ignore the ingredients, however. Instead, start by scanning for a section on the package called "active ingredients." This is where you'll find the most potent chemicals. As for the long list of unpronounceable ingredients, focus at the top. By law, manufacturers must present them in order of concentration. If you want a cleanser with vitamin C or glycolic acid, look for it in the first few items on the list. If you typically steer clear of oil-based products, don't automatically dismiss a lotion if mineral oil is the twentieth ingredient—unless, of course, using it will make you break out. If you have any skin allergies, even the tiniest speck of the offending chemical can cause a reaction, so you should look over the entire package with an eagle eye.

The Game Plan: Six Do-at-Home Steps for Lowering Your SVA

1. Commit to washing your face twice a day. If your skin is extremely dry, wash once, just before going to bed, to dislodge any dirt, oil, makeup, or other residue inside your pores. Not only will this make your skin immediately look more radiant, it will also help any treatment products (including anti-aging creams) that you apply afterward to penetrate and work more effectively while you sleep.

2. Choose the right cleanser. A facial wash shouldn't leave your skin feeling uncomfortably tight, and it shouldn't make your face sting. If your cleanser is too harsh or drying, it will actually increase your SVA. Using my cleanser list as a guide, choose a formula that leaves your skin comfortably tight, but not red, flaky, or irritated.

3. Exfoliate. Periodically removing the top layer of dead skin cells—the layer that is responsible for making complexions look dull—will instantly make you look younger and more radiant. An exfoliant, even more than a cleanser, will help any lotion, serum, or cream you apply afterward penetrate more effectively. Just be careful not to overdo it. Once or twice a week is usually sufficient. If you have very sensitive skin or eczema, you might not be able to exfoliate at all.

4. Read the ingredients. Don't worry about all those unpronounceable names. Just look for the stuff you want: glycolic acid, antioxidants, or aloe, for example. Focus on the beginning of the list, since companies list their ingredients in order of concentration.

5. Know that there is a cleanser for you. You might have to try a few different cleansers at first, but never give up hope of finding the right one for you. With all the new lovely products out there, you will certainly find the one that suits your skin: oily, dry, sensitive, dark, or light.

6. Stay open to change. A cleanser that worked wonders for your skin three months ago might leave your skin flaky or oily now. Whether this is because of a change in seasons or because of a new moisturizer you're using, be adaptable. As soon as you notice that your facial wash isn't doing what it's supposed to do, consult a dermatologist, or my cleanser list, for help in choosing a new formula.

4

Treat

Skin-treatment product is a rather vague term. Since no two people's skin is exactly the same, you can't treat their skin problems exactly the same. Some of my patients want to make their dull complexions more radiant. Others want to minimize fine lines or even out their skin's texture. Some are battling lingering acne, and still others merely want to moisturize their parched-looking cheeks. Which treatment products are exactly right for you? How can you make the most of the wealth of treatment ingredients that are available? Most important, which ones will let you chip away at your SVA without surgery and other in-office treatments? Before we discuss that, let's start with a handful of questions to gauge how much you know about the bottles and tubes you probably have in your bathroom.

1. Most people are better off using some sort of skin-treatment product
   A. Twice a day
   B. At least once a day

C. No more than a few times a week

2. Prescription retinoids, like Retin-A, Renova, and Avage, can help to treat

   A. Acne

   B. Wrinkles

   C. Early signs of skin cancer and both of the above

3. Antioxidants are good tools in the fight against aging because they

   A. Prevent sun damage by mopping up free radicals

   B. Prevent sun damage and also reverse it

   C. Work as sunscreens by blocking UV light

4. Taking oral antioxidants, like green tea, coenzyme Q10, and vitamins C and E, along with eating foods rich in antioxidants, like blueberries, sweet potatoes, and tomatoes

   A. Will probably keep my skin looking young just as much as, if not more than, using topically applied antioxidants

   B. Might keep me healthy but will do nothing for my SVA

   C. Is not very effective

5. If I want to lower my SVA over time, my best bet is to

   A. Use a good-quality moisturizer and a sunscreen

   B. Ask my dermatologist about prescription retinoids

   C. Scrub with an exfoliating cleanser

6. If I want my skin to look younger within seconds, I'm better off

   A. Using a good-quality moisturizer

   B. Relying only on prescription retinoids

   C. Scrubbing with an exfoliating cleanser

7. Cosmeceuticals are

   A. A marketing gimmick

   B. Hybrid products that straddle the line between cosmetics and pharmaceutical prescription creams and lotions

   C. Topical ingredients that mimic the effect of Botox

8. The important thing to know about chemical peels is that
   A. They are dangerous and should be used only to treat very dramatic aging
   B. They all penetrate very deeply, so I will have to plan on going into hiding for a week after having one
   C. They come in a wide variety of strengths, from superficial ones that will allow me to go right back to my daily activities to very deep ones that require a week or more of downtime

9. The good news about acne is that
   A. People with higher SVAs rarely suffer from it
   B. There is a large selection of very effective treatments for every type of acne, from over-the-counter creams and lotions to aggressive prescription medications designed for the most severe cases
   C. The oral prescription drug Accutane works well and is safe for anyone to use, even someone with mild acne

10. Rosacea is
    A. Another form of acne
    B. Not treatable at all, unfortunately
    C. A condition involving broken red blood vessels, flushing, and acnelike pimples that tends to worsen with age

Answers

1. A: I tell all my patients not to let a single twelve-hour period pass without applying some form of treatment ingredients to your skin, whether it's a moisturizer with anti-aging benefits, a good-quality wrinkle cream, or a gentle acne-fighting lotion.

2. C: I call prescription retinoids the gold standard when it comes to reversing and preventing the signs of aging. In addition to treating acne, these vitamin A derivatives help to shed outer cells, replacing them with plumper, healthier, better-arranged ones. They also normalize blood vessels and stimulate the

production of new collagen fibers and hyaluronic acid. Doctors now believe that retinoids can stop (or even reverse) the early signs of skin cancer.

3. A: Although antioxidants can't reverse sun damage or block ultraviolet rays, they do help to prevent injury by neutralizing the damaging free radicals that the skin produces when it is exposed to UV light.

4. A: This is one more reason to take your vitamins and eat your fruits and vegetables. In addition to helping your body function well on the inside, oral antioxidants help to mop up the free radicals in your skin just as effectively as, and possibly *more* effectively than, topically applied antioxidants do.

5. B: Moisturizers hydrate your skin, but without added anti-aging ingredients, they won't help your skin to "behave" as if it's younger. Sunscreens help to prevent sun damage and subsequent skin aging, but they do nothing to reverse existing sun damage. Exfoliating cleansers will restore a youthful radiance to your face, but if you're looking for real, long-term improvement, retinoids are the gold standard.

6. A: If you want instant gratification, apply a good-quality moisturizer, which will immediately plump up fine lines, making them less visible. Just be sure to continue using products that lead to long-term improvement as well, like prescription retinoids.

7. B: Cosmeceuticals are a relatively new breed of over-the-counter skin-care products that offer some of the benefits of prescription formulas, but in weaker concentrations. What really separates cosmeceuticals from prescription items is that the latter require approval from the Food and Drug Administration (FDA)—even topical creams.

8. C: Like anything else, chemical peels *can* be unsafe when they are done by someone who isn't trained or supervised by a doctor. As long as you choose an experienced practitioner, they're

perfectly safe. They come in strengths ranging from very light to quite deep, and they can reveal younger-looking skin with minimal downtime.

9. B: Unfortunately, we're seeing more and more cases of acne among adults. Although Accutane is a highly effective treatment, it's not for everyone—you'll read more about that later. There are many therapies, however—ranging from lotions and creams to pills, lights, and lasers—to ensure that there's help for anyone who needs it.

10. C: Rosacea might look like acne, but the condition—characterized by flushing, broken red blood vessels, and papules and pustules all centered around the cheeks and nose—is actually a completely different phenomenon. Fortunately, with every passing year we're finding better, more effective ways of controlling it.

Alison's Story: The Bride-to-Be

Alison, who is twenty-seven years old, was planning her wedding. She had hired a photographer, a caterer, and a band. Her dress was picked out, and her hairstylist and makeup person were booked. With barely six weeks to go until the big day, the one thing that hadn't been addressed was her skin. From a distance, Alison had a gorgeous, glowing complexion, but up close, I could already see evidence of her sun-worshiping past—and so could Alison. Faint tiny brown spots had begun to mottle her cheeks, three fine horizontal lines cut across her wide forehead, and more tiny lines crept outward from the corners of her eyes when she smiled. Offhand, I'd say that her skin's virtual age was at least five years older than her actual age.

None of this was very obvious to casual observers; clearly, Alison had not been neglecting her skin. Nevertheless, she had fallen under the spell that strikes most brides-to-be. For the past several months, she had pored over wedding magazines and their exhaustive beauty time lines. "Isn't there something I should be doing before the big day?" she kept asking me. I booked a couple of glycolic peels to brighten her face, prescribed a retinoid cream, and gave her some nice skin-care products as a wedding present. Then, after much pleading on her part, I wound up relaxing those forehead lines and her almost invisible crow's feet with a touch of Botox. After all, when you have just six weeks, even the best topicals can accomplish only so much. However, if it's not your goal to look absolutely perfect overnight, a month and a half is plenty of time for creams, lotions, and serums to begin making serious inroads toward lowering your SVA, especially if obvious signs of aging haven't started to appear.

The Importance of Starting a Skin-Care Routine Early

When younger women come to me for the first time, they're typically hoping to give their skin more of a finished, polished look. Here's a typical scenario: A patient has recently graduated from college. She's started her first serious job and has replaced her T-shirts, blue jeans, and flats with tailored skirts and heels. She's found a decent hairstylist and has invested in a good lipstick. After studying the faces of some of the older women at work—or perhaps her mother's face—she has decided that she doesn't want her complexion to go down that same road. It's time, she decides, to invest in her skin, too.

This is a smart idea. It's easy to feel invincible when you look at your smooth, glowing skin in the mirror, but just about the worst thing you can do is to take it for granted. It amazes me how many women go to bed with all of their makeup on after a late night out. Many others don't take the proper amount of time to at least cleanse at the end of a long day; they neglect to use sunscreen and treatment creams and lotions, and they spend their vacations baking on the beach, because, they figure, everything looks good now. Excessive sun exposure, both past and present, is always the biggest concern about skin condition, even though the damage might just be starting to appear. If you don't take action early, it will manifest itself in the form

Myth My skin looks fine, so there is no reason to start a skin-care regimen just yet.

Truth The very best time to start a serious skin-care regimen is when your complexion is at its absolute best. When you don't have to spend your time and money addressing existing problems, you have plenty of energy to focus on preventing problems that might surface later. Furthermore, the earlier you incorporate my simple cleanse-treat-prevent system into your routine—making it as much a part of your day and night as brushing your teeth—the sooner this system will feel so automatic and so instinctive that you'll be amazed you ever lived without it!

of fine lines, brown spots, and possibly skin cancer by your early thirties. Whether you're twenty, thirty, or seventy, it's never too late to adopt a good topical treatment plan and to keep amending it as your complexion ages.

Surface Improvements

If you take one message away from this book, I hope it's this: the key to lowering your SVA at home is not to let any twelve-hour period pass without doing something beneficial for your complexion. In the morning, the number-one action you can take is to wear sunscreen; that should be a no-brainer (see chapter 5). In the evening, it's easy to forget the importance of skin care, especially if your face is clear and free of wrinkles. Perhaps this tip will help you to remember: by applying a treatment product before bed every night beginning tonight, you can start spending your sleeping hours becoming younger-looking instead of older-looking. How's that for an incentive?

It certainly was an incentive for Danielle, a thirty-six-year-old college professor who first came to see me after noticing that her face was slowly beginning to take on the uneven pigmentation and fine lines that she associated with her older sister. She assumed that I was going to push her toward lasers and Botox, and she made it clear that she wasn't ready for those treatments. When I told her that we could come up with a simple regimen of products that are available at her local drugstore, Danielle looked at me incredulously. "You're trying to tell me that I can make a significant difference in my skin simply by applying a lotion or a cream?" she asked, laughing. "It's hard enough to make sense of all the bottles and tubes in the beauty aisle!"

Danielle is right about the second point. Every year brings a slew of new ingredients that are touted for their ability to turn back the clock. Some of them work beautifully; others seem to be more hype than anything else. In this chapter, I've outlined some of the biggies—the ones you're most likely to encounter at the drugstore, the department store counter, and the dermatologist's office—and graded them for proven effectiveness and potency. (Grade A ingredients are among the strongest and most effective, whereas grade C ingredients might be weaker or have very little data to back up the claims manufacturers make.) You can use these ingredients at any age, but if your SVA is more than a few years above your chronological age, it's always a good idea to upgrade to one or more of the aggressive treatments.

Let me start with another story: A thirty-six-year-old patient named Jessica was shopping a few months before her fifteen-year college reunion. She was looking forward to the event, and why shouldn't she? Jessica was a successful executive at a marketing company and the mother of two great kids. She pulled two beautiful cocktail dresses off the rack, walked into the changing room, faced the three-way mirror, and couldn't quite believe what she saw. "My God," she thought, "what's happened to me? Is it just the fluorescent lights, or am I suddenly looking my age?"

Studying her reflection, Jessica noticed that the luster she had always taken for granted in her twenties and early thirties had vanished from her skin. She saw brown spots dotting her cheeks, fine wrinkles around her eyes, and the sharp frown lines between her brows that dermatologists call glabellar creases. Feeling too disheartened and defeated to try on anything, Jessica left the two dresses on the hook, grabbed her purse, and left the store. Back in the comfort and warm lighting of her own bathroom, her skin looked ten times better.

Nevertheless, Jessica had seen the writing on the dressing-room wall, and the next week she was sitting in my office. With her college reunion only three months away, one of the first things she asked me about was Retin-A. She'd been hearing about the product for years—first as a treatment for acne and later as a wonder weapon against wrinkles. However, she had no idea where to find it, or whether it was right for her.

I prescribe topical retinoids like Retin-A to many patients in their thirties, but it's even better to start using them in your twenties. If you've strictly been using over-the-counter alpha hydroxy acids and retinols (weaker cousins of retinoids), you might notice that even though they're great ingredients, they don't impart the same smoothness and glow as they did five or ten years ago. Now is an excellent time to upgrade your treatment regimen.

Here is your first assignment for your bedtime treatment regimen: if you haven't done so already, switch to a nighttime product containing at least one of the ingredients discussed below. (With the exception of prescription retinoids, most of them fall under the term *cosmeceuticals*; although they're available over the counter, they claim to have the benefits of a prescription cream. See the "What Are Cosmeceuticals, Anyway?" sidebar on page 74 for more information.)

If you want to boost your morning regimen as well, look for a sunscreen that is spiked with an item or two from this list or add a separate anti-aging day lotion.

Retinoids

Retinoids are truly the gold standard when it comes to knocking years off your SVA because they reverse and prevent the signs of aging. When a retinoid is applied to the skin regularly, the vitamin A derivatives help to shed the cells of the outer skin layer (the epidermis) that have become flat and jumbled after prolonged sun exposure, replacing them with plumper, healthier, better-arranged cells. Underneath the surface, in the second layer of skin (the dermis), the retinoid normalizes blood vessels and stimulates the production of new collagen fibers and hyaluronic acid. The new fibers replace at least some of the irregular, thick, clumpy, sun-damaged ones. The result is better texture, more even color, and increased radiance in as little as two weeks. After every month and year of a retinoid's use, the improvement only continues. There's even evidence to show that retinoids can stop (and possibly reverse) early signs of skin cancer.

Retin-A has been around since the early 1970s as an acne treatment, but once dermatologists caught on to its anti-aging capabilities, it became very popular as a prescription item for skin aging. The company developed a few variations on the formula, such as Retin-A Micro, a less-irritating form of Retin-A, and Renova, a more moisturizing version, which are highly effective in treating sun damage.

Myth If my skin isn't red and scaly, my treatment product isn't working.

Truth The "no pain, no gain" approach is for marathon training, not skin care. Yet I still meet many women who continue to have facials that leave their complexions looking angry, who insist on using harsh lotions, or who use their prescription retinoid so frequently that they make their faces burn and peel. They tell me that this is how they know the treatment is doing its job. Here's the real scoop: First, you don't need an extra-strong product to make a difference in your skin. For example, studies show that the tried-and-true acne fighter benzoyl peroxide works just as well in 2.5 and 5 percent concentrations as it does in 10 percent concentrations—and the lower concentrations are far less likely to leave an unsightly crust in their wake. Second, by irritating the skin, you're breaking down its protective outer layer, which means that it can't perform as efficiently as it usually does. It also looks pretty crummy. There are, of course, exceptions. In-office procedures like microdermabrasion, peels, and certain lasers are designed to wound the skin mildly to promote collagen production. When you're choosing a product to use at home, however, the ones that feel fabulous going on will leave your skin looking even more fabulous in the end.

Now the prescription retinoid landscape is crowded with more names, like Differin, Avage, and Tazorac. Each is available only by prescription, and each has its own pros, cons, and potential for irritation. In general, the lower concentrations are gentler but less effective, and the gel forms are a bit harsher than the creams. Differin is the least irritating of the group but might also be the least effective. A new 0.3 percent gel has recently been released, and I believe that it works better than the original 0.1 percent, for both acne and photoaging (the cumulative effects of UV exposure). If you are planning to use Differin to treat skin aging, I would recommend the higher concentration. Avage and Tazorac are actually identical formulas under two different prescription names: Tazorac is typically prescribed for psoriasis, and Avage for acne. For most people, both are a bit more irritating than Differin but a bit less irritating than Retin-A. It's best to ask your dermatologist which retinoid is ideal for you. Most will send you home with some samples to try. This way, you can be sure that you can tolerate a product before you pay for an expensive prescription.

You'll notice that retinoids come in many different concentrations. Before automatically asking for the strongest one, remember that it's far better to regularly apply a retinoid that your skin can handle than to choose one so irritating that you won't want to use it at all. My basic rule is the following: to see the fastest, most dramatic improvement, you should use the highest concentration that your skin can tolerate without becoming red and flaky. That often means starting with a weaker retinoid a few times a week, then working your way up to a stronger concentration.

The best time to apply a retinoid is before bedtime, at least five minutes after washing and drying your face. (If you still find the formula irritating, try waiting half an hour after drying your face.) By applying the formula at night, you'll give it eight uninterrupted hours to work its magic without any sun exposure. (Since retinoids make the skin sensitive to the sun, it's best to avoid sun exposure soon after applying a retinoid and be even more obsessive than usual about wearing facial sunscreen while you're using these products.)

Not long ago, a patient named Isabel told me that she adores her Retin-A; then she added that of course she stops using it during the summer in order to avoid excess sun damage. I'm always surprised by how many people believe that they're helping their skin by doing this. Their motivations are admirable, but they're actually making a big mistake by cheating themselves out of two or three months' worth of SVA-lowering opportunities. Unless you are lying in the sun or performing activities in direct sunlight without sunscreen, using Retin-A at bedtime is perfectly safe.

To maximize a retinoid's effectiveness and minimize irritation, wait at least five minutes after washing your face, then squeeze a pea-size amount onto your index finger; more is *not* better in this case. (Retin-A Micro now comes in a pump that dispenses the precise amount.) Place dots of even amounts on the center of your forehead, chin, and each cheek, then blend gently into the skin.

Keep in mind that the retinol you see in nearly every over-the-counter anti-aging product is *not the same* as prescription retinoids. Studies show that retinol has some of the same benefits as a retinoid, but it's not nearly as effective. On the other hand, it's also much less irritating, so for the few of you who cannot tolerate at least one of the prescription retinoids, you can use retinol with abandon. Below are some of my favorite retinol-containing products. (Grade: A)

Dr. Dover Recommends

Drugstore
- Skin Effects Daily Anti-Aging Treatment Cream SPF 15
- Skin Effects Lightweight Moisturizing Soufflé SPF 30
- Olay Total Effects Intensive Restoration Treatment with Pro-Retinol + VitaNiacin
- Neutrogena Healthy Skin Anti-Wrinkle Intensive Night Cream
- RoC Retinol Actif Pur Anti-Wrinkle Night Treatment
- La Roche-Posay Biomedic Retinol 15

Department Store and Doctor's Office

- SkinCare Prescription Night Anti-Aging Moisturizer with Retinol
- SkinMedica Retinol Complex
- SkinCeuticals Retinol 1.0 Maximum Strength Refining Night Cream
- DDF Retinol Energizing Moisturizer
- Murad Skin Perfecting Lotion
- Clé de Peau Intensive Wrinkle Corrective Cream

I hate to see a patient toss her prescription retinoid aside because it made her skin red and flaky. Certainly some people just can't tolerate the ingredient, but it's far more likely that they're using it improperly or not allowing their face to get used to the formula. If your skin becomes red, irritated, or scaly when you apply your retinoid, stop using it immediately. Wait for the irritation to subside, then give it another try, applying it only every second or third night. Be sure to wait until your face is completely dry before rubbing it into your skin, and use it sparingly. This method works for nearly all of my patients. As you get used to the product, slowly increase the frequency of application until you can use it every night or every other night.

If the irritation recurs even after this, your skin is trying to tell you something. The next step is to try a less irritating prescription retinoid; —in most cases your doctor will be able to find one you can tolerate. On the off chance that your face can't handle even the gentlest formula, take heart: your doctor has a wealth of alternatives to offer you.

Alpha Hydroxy Acids

Glycolic, lactic, and fruit acids all fall under the category of alpha hydroxy acids, or AHAs. Blended into topical lotions, these ingredients break down the epidermis, increasing cell turnover and revealing brighter, younger-looking skin underneath, thus offering an effortless way to gradually scale down your skin's virtual age. Higher-concentration formulas produce more skin shedding and speedier results, but they can also cause unwanted peeling and redness, especially if you have sensitive skin. Also keep in mind that AHAs work slowly and subtly. They can help to fade brown spots and fine lines but will never make them go away entirely. (Grade: A)

Dr. Dover Recommends

Drugstore

- Olay Regenerist Daily Thermal Mini-Peel
- Eucerin Plus Intensive Repair Lotion
- La Roche-Posay Biomedic LHA serum

Department Store and Doctor's Office

- SkinCare Prescription Age Reversal Glycolic Acid Serum
- NeoStrata Ultra Daytime Skin Smoothing Cream AHA 10 SPF 15
- Dr. Brandt Laser A-Peel
- SkinCeuticals C + AHA
- DDF Glycolic 10% Exfoliating Moisturizer

Antioxidants

There's a reason that researchers are buzzing about this exciting area of skin science. Antioxidants seem to slowly lower your SVA by helping to prevent free radicals from damaging and aging healthy skin cells. This potentially staves off not only skin cancer but also wrinkles and brown spots. Some of the most promising antioxidants include idebenone (which is in the cream Prevage), coenzyme Q10, vitamins E and C, and botanicals like soy, green tea, malic acid, and pomegranate. Remember that antioxidants prevent sun damage but do not reverse it. Unlike prescription retinoids, which make your skin look younger by reversing sun damage, antioxidants simply prevent further damage. Although they haven't proven to be as effective as retinoids, I still believe that they're an important part of everyone's skin-care regimen, regardless of age. (Grade: A–)

Dr. Dover Recommends

Drugstore

- Skin Effects Intensive Eye Treatment
- Skin Effects Eye Effects Dual Action Under Eye Therapy
- Skin Effects Daily Anti-Aging Treatment Cream SPF 15
- Skin Effects Lightweight Moisturizing Soufflé SPF 30+
- Neutrogena Anti-Oxidant Age Reverse Day Lotion SPF 20
- La Roche-Posay Active C Facial Moisturizer for Normal to Combination Skin

Department Store and Doctor's Office

- SkinCare Prescription Age Prevention Vitamin C Serum
- SkinCare Prescription Intensive Anti-Wrinkle Moisturizer
- SkinCeuticals C E Ferulic Combination Antioxidant Treatment
- SkinCeuticals Serum 10 AOX+
- Prevage Anti-Aging Treatment
- La Mer The Radiant Infusion
- Orlane Extreme Line Reducing Re-Plumping Cream
- La Prairie Cellular Resurfacing Cream
- Dr. Brandt Poreless Moisture
- Cellex-C High Potency Serum
- DDF Silky C Serum
- Murad Essential-C Daily Renewal Complex
- N.V. Perricone M.D. Concentrated Restorative Cream

Peptides

If glycolic acid was the "it" item in the 1990s, peptides are the current ingredient du jour. Peptides are tiny chains of amino acids that make up proteins. The brain's pituitary gland uses peptides as messengers, sending them through the bloodstream to signal the rest of the body to carry out virtually all of its daily functions. Some people believe that when peptides are applied topically, they can prompt the skin cells to make more collagen, the epidermis to normalize, and the blood vessels to become plumper and healthier—all of which should, in theory, reduce your SVA over time. Matrixyl and Dermaxyl are two of the few peptides I've seen that have some really good supporting science behind them to show that they make older skin look younger. Meanwhile, scientists are studying many more peptides, which means that other effective ones will come onto the scene before long. (Grade: A–)

One emerging class of peptides temporarily changes the tone of the facial muscles, relaxing the ones that are responsible for crinkling so that the skin looks smoother and fine lines are less obvious. Some of the latest include GABA, which stands for gamma-aminobutyric acid. This is an interesting compound that is derived from tomatoes and that also contains the potent antioxidant lycopene. You get instant gratification as well as some of the long-term anti-aging benefits of an antioxidant. (Another agent, DMAE, which stands for dimethyl-aminoethanol, is a neurotransmitter that works similarly to GABA to induce temporary smoothing of the skin.)

Ninety percent of my patients who apply one of these skin-smoothing peptides look better ten minutes later. Let me emphasize that this is *not* Botox. Peptides do not stop facial muscles from functioning; they merely relax them for about twelve hours. This is why so many people love them; the results are immediate, short-term, painless, and relatively inexpensive. (Grade: A–)

Dr. Dover Recommends

Drugstore
- Skin Effects Cell 2 Cell Continuous Action Anti-Wrinkle Care
- Skin Effects Targeted Anti-Aging Treatment
- Skin Effects Intensive Overnight Repair Cream
- Skin Effects Wrinkle Relax Serum
- Olay Regenerist Daily Regenerating Serum
- Olay Regenerist Derma-Pod Eye System, Anti-Aging Triple Response

- Olay Regenerist Micro-Sculpting Cream

Department Store and Doctor's Office
- SkinCare Prescription Intensive Anti-Wrinkle Moisturizer
- Dr. Brandt r3p Cream
- La Prairie Cellular Nurturing Complex
- DDF Wrinkle Relax
- Patricia Wexler M.D. Dermatology Intensive 3-in-1 Eye Cream: Lifting, Firming, Anti-Wrinkle Formula
- N.V. Perricone M.D. Neuropeptide Facial Conformer

Copper Peptides

Copper peptides are another class of peptides. There are data to prove that copper peptides make brown spots and wrinkles fade, but the benefit is very slight—not nearly as dramatic as with Retin-A or other retinoids. If the moisturizer you use on top of your retinoid happens to contain copper peptides (along with any of the other ingredients described in this section), it certainly can't hurt. (Grade: B)

Dr. Dover Recommends

Drugstore
- Neutrogena Visibly Firm Face Lotion SPF 20

Growth Factors

First, a little background on growth factors: When epidermal cells are grown in a lab, they produce a serum filled with many of the compounds that are found in healthy newborn skin. These compounds, called growth factors, are responsible for healing wounds and for the production of new skin cells. They are just the kind of ingredients you want on your skin to make it look its best. For a few years, skin-care companies have been packaging this serum into formulas. Made properly, they really do help the skin.

One of the most popular and well-regarded growth factors, TNS Recovery Complex—which many of my patients swear by—has split-face studies: the side of the face that was treated by the serum looks brighter, fuller, and less blotchy and wrinkled and has more healthy color. My biggest objection is that the stuff feels sticky and smells a bit like sweaty socks. One patient told me that she brought it to a brunch and had ten of her girlfriends try it out. They all thought she was a nut and could not believe that she was voluntarily putting such a horrible-smelling serum on her face. On the other hand, many of my patients love the results they see with this growth factor serum and use it faithfully.

Another product, RéVive, which was developed from research performed on burn victims, might work just as well. At $600 per ounce, it should. In 2005, *Forbes* put RéVive on its "Most Expensive Cosmetics" list. There's also a growth factor line sold through doctors' offices called Neocutis. The line includes Journée Bio-restorative Day

Myth The more expensive a face cream, the better it works.

Truth Many skin-care companies want you to think that this is true, so they spend millions of dollars on advertising to coax you into believing it. Although it's very possible that some of those fancy products *will* do wonders for your complexion, you're often also paying for beautiful packaging and the glossy advertising campaigns that lured you in the first place. There are plenty of affordable drugstore skin products that contain effective, high-quality ingredients; indeed, my own line, Skin Effects, which is sold at CVS, uses the same laboratory and the same high-quality ingredients that many of the best "prestige" department-store brands do. For example, the active ingredient in our wrinkle-relaxing product, Wrinkle Effects, is lycopene, the identical ingredient found in the best skin-tightening items that sell for more than five times as much at high-end department stores. Nevertheless, some of my patients have $200-a-jar creams decorating their vanities—and they swear by these potions. Their skin looks great, so I certainly won't argue with them.

Cream, Lumière Bio-restorative Eye Cream, Bio-Gel Bio-restorative Hydrogel, and Hyalis 1% Hyaluronate Refining Serum. All feature a cocktail of growth factors called processed skin cell proteins. Growth factors aren't cheap, no matter what brand you buy. For those who wish to use them and who don't mind shelling out the cash, I recommend applying one as an adjunct to retinoids, not as a substitute for them. (Grade: A–)

Dr. Dover Recommends

Department Store and Doctor's Office
- RéVive Intensité Crème Lustre
- SkinMedica TNS Recovery Complex
- NeoCutis Journée Bio-restorative Day Cream
- NeoCutis Bio-Gel Bio-Restorative Hydrogel
- NeoCutis Hyalis 1% Hyaluronate Refining Serum

Kinetin

This plant-derived hormone was for a long time billed as a nonirritating alternative to retinoids. Companies that make products containing kinetin have claimed that the extract helps to repair damaged skin cells and protect them from further injury—and that it is ideal for those with sensitive or red-toned skin and those with rosacea who cannot tolerate prescription retinoids. However, there's not much data to support these claims. (Grade: B)

Dr. Dover Recommends

Department Store and Doctor's Office
- SkinCare Prescription Intensive Anti-Wrinkle Moisturizer
- Kinerase Cream or Lotion with SPF 30

Oral Supplements

Although the jury's still out on how much oral antioxidants will help your skin's SVA, there's pretty good evidence that ingesting antioxidants could be just as important as rubbing them onto the skin, if not more so. For one thing, taking them by mouth is the only way to ensure that your entire body—including your lungs, liver, and heart—reap the benefit of these powerful compounds.

Eating a well-balanced diet of green, yellow, and orange fruits and vegetables is the best way to fast-track antioxidants into your bloodstream. All contain healthy phytochemicals that dietary supplements do not. Besides, enjoying good food is infinitely more appealing than popping pills, especially given the fact that two of the best antioxidant sources around are red wine and quality dark chocolate. Nevertheless, there are a few oral supplements that I do recommend, based on a Harvard Medical School article that appeared in the *New England Journal of Medicine*. Author and researcher Walter Willett determined that taking a daily multivitamin, extra amounts of vitamins A, B_6, B_{12}, C, D, and E, and calcium is most important for overall health. Anything that promotes overall health certainly promotes skin health. (Grade: A–)

Dr. Dover Recommends
Talk to your doctor about how to put together an oral antioxidant supplement program that's ideal for you.

Beat-the-Clock Cheat Sheet

Whether you want to make a difference in your skin's virtual age tomorrow, whether you're looking for long-term improvement, or whether you want the best of both worlds, there's a treatment plan for you. I've broken down my favorite ingredients into three categories. The first will make your skin look younger literally overnight. The second will yield visible changes within four to six weeks. The third offers long-term improvement that takes at least three months to unfold. If you want to keep things really simple, however, all you really need is a prescription retinoid. Following is an explanation of the three categories.

1. To look younger tomorrow morning. Moisturizing ingredients plump and smooth temporarily by boosting the skin's water content. (Creams tend to give a dewier look than lotions do because they're richer and more hydrating.) Humectants, like glycerin, lactic acid, and hyaluronic acid, draw water from the deeper to the more superficial layers of skin, so they are great tools for moisturizing the skin. They are also a terrific choice for breakout-prone people who can't tolerate oily products. Occlusives, such as petrolatum, work by sealing in the existing moisture and preventing water molecules from evaporating; however, they can make some complexions look greasy and may aggravate acne. In fact, unless your skin is flaky or tight, you might not require any moisturizing ingredients at all. If your skin is a mix of oily and dry, use a light anti-aging lotion over the entire face, then rub a separate moisturizer into the rougher patches.

2. To look younger in four to six weeks. Ingredients that increase cell turnover, like alpha hydroxy acids, will boost the skin's glow and color. I tell my patients, however, that prescription retinoids are truly the gold standard for reversing and preventing the signs of aging. Applied to the skin regularly, retinoids produce increased skin radiance in as little as two weeks, and the improvement only continues over time. (See "Retinoids," earlier in chapter, for the details.)

3. To look younger in three months and beyond. If you've been hearing a great deal about topical antioxidants during the past several years, there's a good reason. In theory, these vitamins and botanical compounds decrease your body's level of free radicals, or unstable oxygen molecules, which can cause oxidative damage and inflammation in living tissue. Many people now believe that free radicals—which are generated by exposure to ultraviolet light, cigarette smoke, and other environmental hazards—partly account for heart disease, cancer, and at least some of the collagen and elastic fiber destruction that makes skin look older. Eating antioxidant-rich foods and taking supplements helps to mop up the free radicals in the body. Many people believe that applying them topically will do the same for the skin. Antioxidants will not reverse existing sun damage, but they can help to prevent further damage. That's why I suggest using them in conjunction with products that reverse sun damage, like prescription retinoids, other vitamins, or alpha hydroxy acids. Although no one has proven that rubbing antioxidants on your face can make you look younger, I say it certainly can't hurt. Therefore, look for at least one of these names in the first half of the ingredient list on a product label: vitamins C and E, coenzyme Q10, idebenone, green or black tea, pomegranate, soy, or grape-derived malic acid.

Samantha's Story: The Power of Topical Products

Topical products are stronger and more effective than ever. Nevertheless, many women in their forties, fifties, sixties, and seventies continue to ask me whether these products can possibly be potent enough to help their skin. The answer is absolutely, and I'll illustrate this with a story about one of my patients. Samantha, a forty-two-year-old woman, hated wearing makeup. Tall and willowy with dark hair and freckles, she had grown up in the Northeast but spent much of her adult life in Los Angeles soaking in the California sun. Samantha recently moved back to New England to raise her children, and she realized that the freckles everyone used to think were cute had morphed into big, blotchy brown spots that made her look years older than her actual age. If she had taken my quiz then, I'm sure her SVA would've been forty-seven or forty-eight.

Samantha happens to be my office assistant. After three months of watching my patients improve dramatically with the cleanse-treat-prevent regimens I had given them, one day she finally asked, "When are you going to suggest some of those creams for me?" Simply covering her blotchy areas with makeup wasn't an option for a low-maintenance type like Samantha, and she wasn't ready for an in-office procedure like a laser treatment or a chemical peel. She wanted a routine she could incorporate into her daily life that would make her skin not only look better but also "behave" better, so I prescribed an easy cleanse-treat-prevent regimen: in the morning, a foaming cleanser followed by a lightening gel and a sunscreen to keep more blotches from emerging; at bedtime, the same lightening gel followed by a night cream that contains retinol and vitamin C.

Within a week, Samantha's face looked brighter—even her mother commented on it. Within six weeks, she started hearing the kinds of raves and compliments that she hadn't heard in decades. Once we knew that she could tolerate those products, we added a prescription retinoid, and I'm sure you can guess what happened next. Less than six weeks after that, her skin looked so much better that I'd say her SVA was already a good few years younger. The brown spots started to lighten, the skin's luster started to return, and the skin tone improved as well.

Topicals surely have the power to change the skin, regardless of the shape it's in, and without ravaging it in the process. The last example I'll leave you with is one of my favorites because it's about a friend who's very close to my family. Carole, a woman in her late sixties who had never had cosmetic surgery in her life—and didn't plan to—was one of the most athletic people I knew. She had spent fifty summers playing competitive golf six days a week. Carole was used to strangers telling her how youthful she looked—until all of a sudden they stopped. The sun, it seemed, had finally caught up with her.

After decades of using only a light night cream a few nights a week, Carole asked me whether there was anything simple and noninvasive that she could do to help her skin. This was years ago, before I knew just how effective topical creams could be, but I put something together: a sunscreen in the morning *and* the afternoon, because of the amount of time she spent outside, and a prescription retinoid every other night (to avoid irritation). I also suggested that in the morning she use a wonderfully rich moisturizing cream containing retinol and vitamin C.

What Are Cosmeceuticals, Anyway?
Can They Really Lower My SVA?

People ask me these two questions every day. The short answer to the second one is "Probably." Here's the long answer. Cosmeceuticals are hybrids that straddle the line between cosmetics and pharmaceutical prescriptions. By definition, pharmaceutical prescriptions alter either the structure or the function of the skin, or both. Cosmeceuticals do not do this; at least, they're not supposed to, but that's where it gets tricky. Certain botanical cosmeceuticals, for instance, scavenge free radicals or slow down melanin production. Peptides purportedly make older cells behave as if they were younger. Growth factors help to promote new skin production. If that doesn't classify it as a drug—an agent that alters the structure or the function of the skin—I don't know what does.

What really separates cosmeceuticals from prescription drugs is that the latter require approval from the FDA—even if the product is just a topical cream. Garnering that approval requires large studies that prove effectiveness and safety and cost millions of dollars. Cosmeceuticals, on the other hand, require limited study at a fraction of the cost. For this reason, many items that might otherwise be considered prescription drugs are produced and sold as cosmeceuticals. This gets them into your hands faster and at a lower cost to you and to the manufacturer; however, some, like the $500 formulas, actually wind up costing *you* more. Cosmeceutical labels and advertisements use wording that tiptoes around the FDA rules. They might claim that a cream makes wrinkles or brown spots *appear* less noticeable rather than stating that it *makes* them less noticeable. If a company made that claim, it would be considered a structural change in skin, and that is not allowed under the FDA rules. Companies occasionally cross the line, and the FDA might challenge them, requiring that the label be changed or that the advertisement be dropped altogether.

In fact, many of these products work quite well and have been a boon to thousands of my patients. Ironically, most companies that make cosmeceuticals don't provide the type of research that would prove just how effective the product is for fear of having their over-the-counter best sellers reclassified as prescription drugs.

Given how severe her sun damage was, I didn't expect dramatic or rapid improvement. Nevertheless, after about six weeks her skin started to perk up, and in the next six months it went from looking doughy, pasty, and puffy to looking pinker and brighter, with much more luster. Other board-certified dermatologists were actually asking me what fancy procedures I had done for Carole. Even my wife, Tania, who is also a dermatologist, couldn't get over the change.

In the past six years Carole's skin has continued to improve, and every time I see her I am amazed at how well she has done, with nothing but good skin care. It did take awhile for Carole's complexion to come around, I admit. Generally the older your SVA, the more patient you'll have to be with topicals, and you can always turn to lasers and other more aggressive treatments to speed up the process. I always love retelling this story, however, because it represents the point at which I became a true believer in the power of good skin care at any age.

Moisturizers with Anti-Aging Benefits

When I get onto my soapbox about night treatments, many of my patients say, "But Dr. Dover, I already use a moisturizer before bed— isn't that enough?" Sorry, but it's not—not if you want to change your skin's virtual age for the better. No matter how many hundreds of dollars your night cream costs, and no matter how much it improves the skin's appearance temporarily, it will do very little to stave off wrinkles and brown spots in the long run unless it contains anti-aging ingredients. Those one-trick-pony creams might have been fine for our mothers' or grandmothers' generation, because, frankly, that's all they had.

Today, however, there are so many multitasking moisturizers available—packed with alpha hydroxy acids, vitamins, and other goodies to help repair the skin overnight—that there's no reason to use a stand-alone hydrating cream. Here's my favorite reason to use one of these: they work. Why use a moisturizer *and* an anti-aging cream when you can find one product that does double duty? Some of my favorites even have sunscreen built into them.

Dr. Dover Recommends

Drugstore

- Skin Effects Intensive Overnight Repair Cream
- Skin Effects Hand Rejuvenating Treatment
- Skin Effects Firming Face and Neck Cream
- Skin Effects Daily Anti-Aging Treatment Cream SPF 15
- Skin Effects Lightweight Moisturizing Soufflé SPF 30
- Skin Effects Cell 2 Cell Continuous Action Anti-Wrinkle Care
- Skin Effects Daily Anti-Aging Body Lotion SPF 30+
- Olay Regenerist UV Defense Regenerating Lotion
- Olay Regenerist Deep Hydration Regenerating Cream
- Olay Definity Penetrating Foaming Moisturizer
- Aveeno Active Naturals Daily Moisturizer
- Aveeno Active Naturals Eczema Care Moisturizing Cream
- Aveeno Active Naturals Positively Radiant Daily Moisturizer
- RoC Age Diminishing Moisturizing Night Cream
- Vichy Normaderm Anti-Imperfection Hydrating Care

Department Store and Doctor's Office

- SkinCare Prescription Day Anti-Aging Moisturizer AHA with SPF 15
- Dr. Brandt Liquid Synergy
- Cellex-C Skin Firming Cream Plus
- RéVive Moisturizing Renewal Cream
- DDF Retinol Energizing Moisturizer
- Kinerase Ultimate Day Moisturizer
- SkinMedica TNS Ultimate Daily Moisturizer + SPF 20
- N.V. Perricone M.D. Neuropeptide Firming Moisturizer
- La Mer The Concentrate
- La Prairie Anti-Aging Stress Cream

- Orlane Anti-Wrinkle After-Sun Balm for the Face SPF 15
- SkinMedica TNS Ultimate Daily Moisturizer + SPF 20

In-Office Treatments to Improve Texture

To smooth fine lines, brighten up the skin a bit, and pare down their SVA more quickly, many of my patients supplement their arsenal of topicals with an occasional in-office peel or a series of microdermabrasions. Both lift away dead skin cells the way many anti-aging lotions, creams, and serums do, but they are more aggressive, which means that a single treatment can yield the same results as several weeks or months of home topical treatments. Since these therapies come in a wide range of strengths, they're a great choice for anyone—whether twenty-two years old or seventy-two years old—who wants to give her at-home regimen a booster shot. There is one caveat: if you're using topical prescription retinoids, keep in mind that these procedures will irritate your skin a bit more that they otherwise would if you weren't applying retinoids. It's best to discontinue the retinoid cream at least a few days before each peel or dermabrasion. Following is a description of each technique.

Chemical Peels

Chemical peels use an acid solution to remove the upper layers of the skin and enhance the deeper layers. Just how much you remove, and thus how long you will need to recover, varies tremendously, depending on which type of treatment you and your doctor choose. The deepest peel (called a phenol peel) is reserved for the most sun-damaged, severely wrinkled patients. The phenol peel can reduce deep wrinkles, especially the vertical ones around the mouth, along with brown spots, but after the procedure the skin must be covered in either petroleum jelly or in bandages until a new, bright layer emerges about a week later. Your skin remains sensitive for several more days, and you're usually ready to resume normal activities a week or two after the procedure. (Side effects can include pigment changes and permanent skin lightening or even whitening.)

Phenol peels are very aggressive and have significant potential for side effects. They have become far less popular over the past decade since the development of many safe and highly effective laser and light treatments. Medium-depth, or trichloracetic acid (TCA), peels offer a slightly gentler way to treat lines and pigmentation. The skin peels off over the course of about a week, and the peel leaves the skin sensitive for a week or two longer. TCA peels are still fairly popular—my practice performs quite a few of them. Generally, they come with about a week of downtime. A brown film of altered skin forms within a day of the peel; about four to seven days later it peels off, similar to the way that skin peels off after a sunburn. On the upside, a single TCA peel makes a big difference in the color and tone of the skin, which is a huge advantage for those who don't want to return—or spend the money—for a series of laser or light treatments.

By far, the most popular peels in our office are superficial peels done with glycolic acid. The strongest ones use an unbuffered solution. (Buffered peels suppress the active part of the acid molecule; unbuffered ones do not, making the peels gentler and less uncomfortable but also less effective.) Unbuffered peels sting a bit because they alter the top layer of the skin (the epidermis), but they do a good job of lightening brown spots, smoothing fine lines, brightening the skin, and making lasting improvements in its structure. Most patients opt for 20 to 70 percent unbuffered glycolic peels. These leave the epidermis intact, even out the skin tone, and still leave behind a healthy glow. To maintain the results, I'll often build up the strength slowly, over the course of several peels spaced a few weeks apart.

For a gentler, more pampering experience, I refer patients to our aestheticians. The peels they perform are always buffered and never use concentrations as high as those used by doctors. The decrease in your SVA is less dramatic, and the results aren't as long-lasting, either. Then again, individuals who have a peel performed by our aestheticians enjoy an hour of comfort, have an experience like being in a spa with soothing background music, and leave with the benefit of an effective gentle glycolic peel.

Microdermabrasion

This treatment gently "sandblasts" the skin using a fine spray of aluminum oxide or salt crystals. Microdermabrasion that is administered or supervised by a doctor tends to be more aggressive than the spa procedures that are performed by aestheticians, but not always. The treatment involves little risk and is usually given in a series of six, spaced two to four weeks apart. Although microdermabrasion is primarily done to brighten and polish the skin, it produces changes in the skin on a level similar to those of glycolic peels—and some of the changes are likely to be permanent if the procedure is done aggressively. Regular treatments will keep the complexion looking healthy and bright. I usually see the best results in young skin—the kind with just a few light brown spots and fine or no wrinkles. The more wrinkly and saggy and blotchy the skin is, the less improvement you'll notice.

Vibradermabrasion

Like microdermabrasion, this in-office procedure works by removing layers of dead and damaged skin cells, revealing a younger, brighter complexion underneath and encouraging collagen growth. Because this technique uses textured, gently vibrating paddles rather than aluminum oxide or salt crystals, any resulting redness and swelling is minimal, which makes it an especially good choice for sensitive skin.

Home Improvements

Even if you can barely make time to come in for yearly checkups, let alone follow up with biweekly or monthly glycolic peels or microdermabrasion, you can still make a fast, noticeable difference in your skin's virtual age. The latest home kits let you set up shop in your own bathroom, offering an excellent alternative to in-office procedures, as long as the kits are made by companies that are known and respected for their skin-care products. (Increasing numbers of dermatologists are also creating kits.) Home kits are typically quite mild, and by law, home peel kits must self-neutralize to prevent burning the skin. (On the other hand, they yield less improvement than in-office treatments do.)

This doesn't mean that you should use them recklessly. Resist the temptation to peel or sandblast your face more frequently than the directions call for, or you'll risk irritation—especially if you've been using harsh lotions or creams regularly. I also recommend cutting back on the prescription retinoids for a week before doing a home procedure.

Dr. Dover Recommends

Drugstore

- Skin Effects Skin Renewal System Micro Peel Kit
- Olay Regenerist Microdermabrasion and Peel System
- Olay Regenerist Daily Thermal Mini-Peel
- La Roche-Posay Biomedic Pre-Peel LHA Solution
- Neutrogena Advanced Solutions At Home MicroDermabrasion System
- L'Oreal Dermo-Expertise Advanced Revitalift Anti-Aging Glycolic Mini Peel Kit
- Vichy Peel Microdermabrasion Rejuvenating Resurfacing Kit

Department Store and Doctor's Office

- SkinMedica Illuminize Peel
- SkinMedica Vitalize Peel
- Dr. Brandt Laser A-Peel
- Patricia Wexler M.D. Dermatology 2-Step Exfoliating Glyco Peel for Acne
- Dr. Brandt Microdermabrasion
- Patricia Wexler M.D. Dermatology Resurfacing Microdermabrasion System
- La Prairie Cellular 3-Minute Peel

Acne

It hardly seems fair: here you are reading about how to prevent wrinkles, and you're more worried about that throbbing pimple emerging on your chin. If your skin's virtual age is higher than you'd like it to be, why are you dealing with such an adolescent problem? Acne is a problem that most people associate with teenagers, but unfortunately, the condition can linger well into your twenties and thirties and even keep cropping up long after. I frequently see patients who make it through adolescence and their college years with nary a blackhead only to find themselves battling pimples as adults, especially during or after pregnancy. Later, as menstrual periods become irregular during perimenopause, fluctuating hormone levels can also result in acne flares. This happens mostly to women who have had acne in the past, but we also see it in those who have always had clear complexions.

Myth My friend's prescription acne product works on her skin, so I can just borrow hers.

Truth This can actually be a good idea with over-the-counter products. Some of my patients have borrowed their friends' topical prescription creams to see how they like them, then they come to me for their own prescription. Keep in mind, however, that topicals take at least ten days to start working, so you won't be able to gauge a product's effectiveness by using it for a mere weekend. *Never* share oral acne medications like antibiotics. Accutane can have dire side effects, especially if you happen to be pregnant.

My acne patients tend to be well-groomed, attractive women in their twenties and thirties who feel overwhelmed and depressed by the uncontrollable state of their skin. At a time in their lives when they should be enjoying life and having fun, they tell me that they look for any excuse not to go out. They walk into my office with downcast eyes and tell me that when they go to meetings, they often race into the conference room first so that they can sit with their most blemished side facing away from the crowd.

I typically see two types of adult acne. The first might appear as only one to three pimples at a time. Although that might seem like no big deal, I have scores of patients who will tell you otherwise. Mia was visibly distraught and quite embarrassed when I examined her face for the first time. She had only a couple of active pimples along her jawline, but they were fairly large and quite tender—the type that tend to last for weeks no matter what kind of over-the-counter treatment you use. Even worse, Mia had a constellation of dark spots in places where blemishes had healed but had never disappeared completely. (I suspect that she had attempted to squeeze some of them.)

On the other end of the spectrum, there are patients like Wendy, a very successful hair colorist who recently walked into my office with her face covered by about twenty pimples of various sizes. She was very perky and pretty—you could tell that she'd look beautiful if she could just clear up her skin. I started by asking about her daily regimen. She had tried the Proactiv system she'd seen advertised on TV and had seen some initial improvement in her smaller pimples, but nothing that really helped her larger, tender spots. Her complexion eventually became red and irritated from overcleansing, so she abandoned all her acne products except for a salicylic acid cleanser that she used twice a day. Fortunately, she wasn't ready to abandon hope.

For Mia, Wendy, or anyone else to begin clearing her acne, it helps to understand what acne is. This skin disorder is incredibly common—so common that it almost seems odd to consider it a disease. Except for the pimples that might appear on a baby's face right after birth, acne doesn't rear its ugly head until puberty, when tiny sebaceous glands, or pores, become much larger. Sebum is the oil that makes skin feel soft and lustrous. It usually drains from the glands in a fine film, but sometimes it becomes trapped inside the pore, expanding it and causing a little bump called a *comedo* (plural, *comedones*). Comedones that remain open are called blackheads; those that close and form a white or yellowy tip are called whiteheads.

The bacteria that normally grow in the skin begin to feed off the gunk that is trapped inside the pore. As these bacteria multiply, they cause inflammation. Some people never get beyond the blackhead or whitehead stage, whereas others are more prone to large red pimples or even bigger, more inflamed nodules that occasionally rupture and become cystic acne. Although many of my teen patients get all these at once, adults usually see the bigger red lesions. These are notoriously difficult to treat: first, because they are large and deep-seated, and second, because adult skin simply tends to be drier and more sensitive than younger skin and doesn't respond to acne treatments as well as teenage skin does. Although banishing pimples might not reduce your skin's virtual age, using harsh medicine to fight it can easily make you look far older than you actually are.

Enough doom and gloom. The good news is that we now have many highly effective nonirritating weapons with which to battle even the most stubborn acne. To help my patients learn about the myriad treatments available, I give them the following list, arranged from most commonly used to least commonly used:

- Topical over-the-counter products like salicylic acid and benzoyl peroxide

- Topical prescription antibiotic creams that keep pores clear and kill bacteria, used along with retinoids

  The first course of treatment is usually a topical one that involves a comedolytic agent to open pores and break out the trapped plug inside; this is used with an antibiotic to kill the bacteria that worsen acne. Excellent comedolytics include retinoids like Retin-A, which is the same prescription ingredient we use to prevent the signs of aging, and benzoyl peroxide, which is available both over-the-counter and by prescription.

  Benzoyl peroxide is one of the best bacteria fighters. Topical prescription antibiotics, like clindamycin, are also quite effective. A great multipronged approach might be Retin-A at bedtime and benzoyl peroxide along with an antibiotic lotion in the morning. For those whose skin can handle it, I might add a wash containing salicylic acid (another comedolytic) once or twice a day.

- Oral antibiotics and hormonal medications, like birth control pills

  Oral antibiotics, like tetracycline, minocycline, doxycycline, and erythromycin, work better than topical versions because they zap bacteria from the inside out and are also anti-inflammatory. They're prescribed slightly less frequently than creams and lotions are, because many of our patients prefer to avoid pills if they can.

Oral antibiotics work best when used in conjunction with topical benzoyl peroxide and prescription retinoids. Although there is some concern that bacteria can build up a resistance to them, this does not appear to be a significant issue. Patients are occasionally worried that antibiotics might interfere with their oral contraceptive pill, but this is also not a real clinical problem.

Shifting hormonal levels can increase both oil production and acne. If pimples increase with ovulation or just before your period, your dermatologist might prescribe oral contraceptives—especially those that are low in progesterone—to even out the monthly fluctuations. Spironolactone, a blood-pressure medication that also reduces the body's quantity of male hormones (which even women have in small amounts), can help as well. See a reproductive endocrinologist if your acne is accompanied by absent or irregular periods, excess facial and body hair, and obesity. These could be symptoms of a treatable hormonal disorder like polycystic ovary syndrome.

- Accutane

  When conventional acne creams and pills don't work, Accutane is usually the last recourse. Within weeks, this drug opens pores, dries out the skin by shrinking the sebaceous glands, and probably also has some anti-inflammatory benefits. Sixty percent of those with severe acne who take Accutane for four to six months never have acne again, which means that the drug has been a true cure. Unfortunately, Accutane comes with potential side effects that range from annoying to serious. Besides resulting in dry skin and chapped lips (some doctors now prescribe very low "maintenance" doses that don't cause this), Accutane can cause depression as well as severe birth defects if you take it while you're pregnant. (Women must use two forms of contraception and take regular pregnancy tests to ensure that they do not become pregnant during treatment.) That's why dermatologists reserve Accutane for only the most stubborn, unrelenting cases, including the type of cystic acne that typically leaves permanent scars.

The Great Light Way

When Wendy, the hair colorist, refused to take Accutane for her persistent acne, I wound up treating her with our traditional treatment pyramid: Retin-A, benzoyl peroxide, an oral antibiotic, and a laser called the Smoothbeam. After two treatments, we saw some improvement; after six, her skin had totally cleared, and two years later it remains that way. Wendy is beaming!

It sounds like science fiction, but infrared lasers like the Smoothbeam, CoolTouch, and Aramis have proven to cause at least a temporary shrinkage of the sebaceous glands. (However, some studies are beginning to question just how effective they are.) Other lasers and colored light sources, when absorbed by the skin, appear to kill surface bacteria. More and more doctors are attempting to amplify the effects of these devices by treating the skin beforehand with a topical gel that enhances light absorption; this is called photodynamic therapy, or PDT, and it kills bacteria *and* shrinks oil glands at the same time. In short, light-based acne procedures have yielded some success stories, but the results are quite uneven and the treatments are expensive.

Another promising acne treatment is the Isolaz PPX system, a painless treatment that uses gentle suction to open the pores and clean out sebum and clogs. Furthermore, Isolaz exposes the skin to intense pulsed light, which reduces skin inflammation and kills pimple-causing bacteria. The treatment is very effective for blackheads, larger blemishes, and, occasionally, cystic acne. Stayed tuned: scientists are developing new ways to battle this frustrating disorder all the time.

If you're curious, ask your dermatologist about these treatments. If he or she can refer you to patients who are happy with their outcomes, you might consider giving one of these methods a try. However, if you see no improvement after the second round, it is probably time to cut your losses and return to more aggressive conventional treatments.

Dr. Dover Recommends

Drugstore

- Skin Effects Acne Treatment System
- Olay Total Effects 7-in-1 Anti-Aging Moisturizer-Plus Blemish Control

- Neutrogena Complete Acne Therapy System
- Aveeno Active Naturals Clear Complexion Daily Moisturizer

Department Store and Doctor's Office
- NeoStrata Acne Spot Treatment Gel, Acne Treatment Solution Pads, and Blemish Treatment Gel
- SkinMedica Acne Treatment, Toner, and Purifying Masque
- Murad Acne Complex Kit
- Murad Post-Acne Spot Lightening Gel
- Patricia Wexler MD Dermatology Anti-Acne Starter Kit
- Proactiv Solution

Available Online Only
- Rodan + Fields Unblemish

Rosacea

When is acne not acne? When pimples are accompanied by flushing and broken blood vessels, the proper diagnosis might be rosacea. Some people begin to notice that the minor facial flushing they experienced in their twenties becomes more pronounced during their thirties and beyond. Although only a dermatologist can make the call, you can look for some telltale signs. True rosacea develops slowly, over several years, and is characterized by easy flushing, chronic redness on the cheeks and nose, and broken blood vessels. Since those who have the disorder also often wind up developing acnelike papules and pustules, it's sometimes called acne rosacea even though it has nothing to do with acne.

There's much we don't know about this frustrating condition, but here's what we have determined: rosacea runs in families, and even though a cure is still in the future, a good dermatologist can help you to minimize the symptoms and slow the condition's progression. When possible, avoid anything that causes blood vessels to repeatedly open and close, like exposure to the heat of the sun, overly vigorous exercise, strong or irritating skin products, steaming hot drinks, spicy foods, and red wine. (Cheap red wines are especially insidious, so why not enjoy one glass of the good stuff instead of several of a so-so variety?) MetroGel, Finacea, and other prescription topicals can be very effective at taming papules and pustules, and so can the oral antibiotics tetracycline, minocycline, and doxycycline.

You can also find a wealth of reasonably priced redness-combating gels and creams at the local drugstore. Some of the most effective ingredients are mineral-rich red algae, which reduces flushing and inflammation; licorice extract; feverfew; and chamomile. Although they don't work nearly as well as more aggressive treatments like lasers and light sources (see "The Great Light Way," on page 85), these formulas are definitely worth a try. I often advise my patients to use them in conjunction with in-office treatments.

The only way to treat broken blood vessels and redness is with a series of laser and other light-source treatments—and they are incredibly effective. Since these can be costly and are not procedures that you necessarily want to do every year, it's especially important afterward to minimize exposure to the triggers listed above in order to help to prevent the symptoms from coming back.

Dr. Dover Recommends

Drugstore
- Skin Effects Redness Control Calming Gel Cleanser
- Skin Effects Redness Control Laser Correcting Treatment
- Skin Effects Redness Control Daily Moisturizer SPF 30+
- Olay Definity Correcting Protective Lotion with SPF 15
- Eucerin Redness Relief Anti-Aging Serum
- La Roche-Posay Rosaliac Anti-Redness Moisturizer
- Aveeno Active Naturals Ultra-Calming Daily Moisturizer with UVA/UVB Sunscreen
- Lubriderm Seriously Sensitive Lotion for Extra Sensitive Dry Skin

Department Store
- Dr. Brandt Pore Effect
- Murad Redness Therapy Recovery Treatment Gel

Why Acne Happens

Good medicine does a lot to improve the majority of acne cases. However, if you're part of the minority that doesn't respond well, you should start to examine your daily habits for clues. After all, every other day you read some report claiming that French fries, exercise, sex, chocolate, dairy products, wheat, mystery "toxins," and anxiety can cause pimples. Is it just me, or are you too feeling anxious just reading this list? Rather than driving yourself crazy with everything you might be doing wrong, familiarize yourself with the handful of culprits that I think might have some validity.

Diet

For years, the party line among dermatologists was that French fries—not to mention milk, butter, and chocolate—had nothing to do with acne. There were simply no studies to back up the link. Nevertheless, I always told patients that if they knew that a particular food, even something as common as crackers, made their skin flare up, don't eat it. Recently, however, a friend and colleague, dermatologist Bill Danby of Dartmouth Medical School, showed that dairy products might indeed cause or aggravate acne. Just remember that the evidence supporting this is hardly conclusive. Some of my patients have stopped eating, butter, cheese, yogurt, milk, and ice cream and have had fantastic results. If you want to try this, do it for two to three months (but take a calcium and vitamin D supplement) and then determine whether your skin is truly any better. If you see no change, there's no sense in depriving yourself.

Stress

In 2003, Stanford University's department of dermatology tracked twenty-two college students during exam and nonexam periods and had some subjects fill out questionnaires rating their stress levels. Even after accounting for changes in diet and number of hours of sleep, the researchers found a correlation between higher stress and more severe acne. That doesn't prove anything definite, but there is no doubt in my mind that stress worsens many skin diseases, especially those on the face. I have sent patients with recurring herpes (cold sores) and eczema to a local clinic that works on the psyche and the skin, with very positive results. If anxiety-reducing techniques such as hypnosis and behavior modification work for those skin disorders, why not for acne?

Cosmetics

Skin-care products and makeup containing oil and other comedogenic (acne-provoking) agents certainly contribute to clogged pores and what dermatologists call acne cosmetica. There's no huge shocker there. However, when is the last time you thought about the goop you put in your hair? Conditioners, hair spray, and pomade are typically very rich in moisturizers and other sticky ingredients. During a sweaty jog, these products can seep down past your scalp, causing breakouts around your forehead and temples. Also, consider whether the pimples on your cheeks and jawline could come from the fact that you're sleeping on sections of your hair every night. I tell my patients to tie back their long hair at night and at the gym (wearing a sweatband just above the hairline can also help) and to wash the face with a really good cleanser immediately after working out.

Please Don't Squeeze!

Believe me, I know how tempting it is to operate on those big, plump pimples and whiteheads in front of your bathroom mirror. I also know that some so-called skin experts say that it's okay to pop the ones that look like they're coming to a head. However, unless the goop inside drains out the second you touch it, all that squeezing and squishing is likely to make things worse. Some of the pus and dead skin cells come out, but much of it is squeezed sideways into the skin through the weakened acne cyst wall, and this leads to swelling, redness, and a brown spot that can last for months—or even to a permanent scar.

Having an aesthetician aggressively extract your blemishes isn't any wiser, no matter how pristine and A-list his or her spa is. Just think: if one out of every ten extractions creates a long-lasting red spot—and your facialist squeezes ten pimples per week—you could have fifty-two lasting marks on your face after one year. There's nothing like permanent, pitted scarring to boost your skin's virtual age. I tell my patients to take the easy road: get some good acne medicines and let them do the work for you. Dabbed on twice a day, benzoyl peroxide is the only ingredient I've seen that's been proven to make existing pimples go away. If you must get rid of a cyst immediately, see a dermatologist you trust for a cortisone injection. The spot will all but disappear within two to three days. At the very least, see an experienced aesthetician recommended by your doctor who knows to only open "ripe" pustules rather than dig away at the skin. An even better option is the Isolaz system, which uses light suction to remove clogs from pores, ensuring that none of the gunk is forced back into the skin and causes unnecessary trauma.

Lightening Pigmentation

Using home remedies to deal with pigmentation problems (such as applying fresh lemon juice to freckles to help fade them safely and gently) will get you nowhere fast. Fortunately, there are plenty of topicals that help fade to pigment safely but *very* gradually. Prescription retinoids will dramatically lighten lentigines (sun-induced brown spots) in one to two years. Glycolic acid products will take even longer. Using them in combination, one in the morning and the other in the evening, gives you the best of both worlds.

Melasma, the brown patches that emerge on the cheeks, forehead, upper lip, and bridge of the nose, often after the hormonal changes associated with pregnancy or oral contraceptive use, responds best to Tri-Luma, a prescription cream that contains 4 percent hydroquinone (which slows production of the skin pigment melanin), Retin-A, and a topical steroid. Although the triple-ingredient cream works best, hydroquinone alone can also help, especially when used at the 4 percent prescription dose. (The 2 percent–strength hydroquinone concentrations offered over the counter are less effective.) The FDA is considering removing hydroquinone from the market, based on circumstantial evidence that it might be carcinogenic. The drug has been unavailable in Europe for years.

As for the slew of other over-the-counter ingredients that claim to lighten pigmentation (such as soy, kojic acid, and licorice root), none of them is as effective as hydroquinone. For those who want a far more aggressive approach, lasers and light sources can erase most sun-induced brown spots in a single treatment, but melasma is much more difficult to treat.

Dr. Dover Recommends

Drugstore
- Skin Effects Advanced Brightening Complex
- Skin Effects Eye Effects Dual Action Under Eye Therapy
- Aveeno Active Naturals Positively Radiant Eye Brightening Cream
- La Roche-Posay Mela-D Skin Lightening Daily Lotion

Department Store
- Dr. Brandt Laser Lightening Day Lotion
- DDF Intensive Holistic Lightener
- Kinerase Brightening Anti-Aging System
- Murad Lighten and Brighten Eye Treatment
- Patricia Wexler M.D. Dermatology Under-Eye Brightening Cream
- La Prairie The Radiance Collection
- La Mer The Radiant Facial
- RéVive Blanche Whiten, Lighten, Brighten

The Game Plan: Six Do-at-Home Steps for Lowering Your SVA

1. Heed the twelve-hour rule. The most efficient way to knock down your skin's virtual age at home is not to let a single twelve-hour period pass without using some sort of topical treatment, whether it's your sunscreen in the morning, a retinoid at night, or simply a moisturizer with anti-aging benefits.

2. Make friends with a retinoid. These prescription vitamin A derivatives are the gold standard when it comes to anti-aging creams. Used properly and started gradually, these topical powerhouses can be used by almost anyone. If you're one of the few whose sensitive skin can't tolerate a retinoid, be sure to incorporate at least one of my favorite SVA-lowering ingredients, like alpha hydroxy acids, peptides, and antioxidants, into your daily and nightly routine (See pages 63–70 for more on these ingredients.)

3. Eat your way to a better SVA. Antioxidants don't come in topical form only. Studies show that the oral forms help to keep the skin looking younger just as effectively, if not more so. That means taking vitamin supplements and consuming plenty of berries (blueberries, raspberries, strawberries, and blackberries), broccoli, tomatoes, red grapes, spinach, green tea, carrots, soy, and whole grains.

4. Protect as you treat. Today's at-home topical treatments work very well—so well that once you've noticed a significant change in your SVA, it's easy to rest on your laurels and forget that your skin will continue to age without the proper precautions. That's why it's crucial to continue using sunscreen every single day to help stave off future brown spots, fine lines, and overall dullness.

5. Go the extra mile. If you want to kick-start your at-home regimen with something more powerful, consider asking your dermatologist about in-office treatments like chemical peels, microdermabrasion, and vibradermabrasion. All lift away the upper layers of the skin, revealing the newer layers below and speeding up collagen production far more dramatically than any topical serum, lotion, or cream can do. Many of these treatments are so gentle that you can resume your normal activities the very same day.

6. Go easy on your pimples. Acne can strike well after your teenage years have ended. Resist battling it with harsh pimple creams and cleansers that will only increase your SVA by making your skin flaky and irritated. Instead, begin at the bottom of my acne-treatment pyramid, starting with the mildest possible therapies and working your way up to the strongest.

5

Prevent

The cliché is that prevention is the best medicine, and when it comes to the sun's damaging rays, truer words have never been spoken. I'm not exaggerating when I say that the vast majority of my patients who are bothered by their high SVAs could have staved off those fine lines, wrinkles, and brown spots simply by shielding their skin more from ultraviolet light: avoiding the sun during its peak hours, liberally applying sunscreen before venturing outside, and shunning tanning beds. Although cleansers, lotions, and creams are tremendously effective in fighting these signs of aging, it's far easier to help to keep those wrinkles and spots from cropping up in the first place. Every person on the planet should practice good sun protection. Before determining what will work for *your* complexion, you have to familiarize yourself with exactly which techniques, ingredients, and products work and which don't. Take the following quiz to measure your sun-protection IQ:

1. When is tanning considered safe?

   A. If I have darker skin to begin with

   B. If I go to a tanning booth that filters out certain types of ultraviolet light

   C. Any tan or burn is an injury to the skin that leads to skin aging and even skin cancer down the road

2. To minimize UV damage to my skin, I should

   A. Apply sunscreen, minimize exposure during the sunniest hours of the day, and wear protective clothing and a hat whenever possible

   B. Swap all my outdoor activities for indoor ones

   C. Get a good healthy tan every spring and before sunny holidays at a tanning booth to give me protection from the sun's rays

3. Which UV rays can penetrate window glass?

   A. UVA rays

   B. UVB rays

   C. Neither one—glass filters out all the sun's damaging rays

4. The SPF number printed on sunscreen bottles refers to how well the formula shields against

   A. All UV light

   B. UVA light only

   C. UVB light only

5. Most people wear

   A. Too little sunscreen

   B. Too much sunscreen

   C. Just about the right amount of sunscreen

6. The deadliest form of skin cancer is

   A. Melanoma

   B. Squamous cell carcinoma

   C. Basal cell carcinoma

7. Why are self-tanning lotions great?

   A. The bronzy color they leave behind protects the skin from ultraviolet light.

   B. They leave a sun-kissed glow without injuring the skin the way that UV rays do.

   C. Both of the above

8. An example of a physical sunblock ingredient is

   A. Avobenzone

   B. Benzophenone

   C. Zinc oxide

9. Sun exposure is the leading culprit behind

   A. Wrinkles

   B. Crow's feet

   C. Brown spots

   D. All of the above

10. You can increase your protection from UV light by supplementing your sunscreen with

    A. Antioxidants

    B. Retinoids

    C. A good moisturizer

Answers

1. C: A tan or a burn, no matter how mild, is a skin injury that can certainly lead to brown spots, fine lines, wrinkles, and even skin cancer years from now, no matter what color your skin is. As for tanning salons that claim to filter out dangerous UV light, don't believe it. Baking there is just as harmful—maybe more so— than baking on the beach.

2. A: I wouldn't give up my favorite outdoor activities, nor should you. Instead, I suggest liberally applying sunscreen every few hours that you're outside and wearing sun-protective clothing, including a hat. When possible, seek the shade during the sunniest hours of the day, from 10 A.M. to 2 or 3 P.M.

3. A: UVA rays, which are responsible for premature aging and skin cancer, travel right through window glass, so wear sunscreen, even when you know you'll spend all day driving in a car.

4. C: A sunscreen's SPF measures only its level of protection from UVB, the rays that cause burning and tanning and can lead to skin cancer later. Formulas labeled "broad spectrum" guard against both UVB *and* UVA. Presently there is no number on a sunscreen bottle for UVA protection, but it's coming soon. In the meantime, be sure that the sunscreen you use contains both UVB and UVA sunscreen agents.

5. A: Studies show that an SPF 30 sunscreen, applied in the quantities most people use, yields an SPF of only about 2! If you apply a great sunscreen liberally, it screens out 98 percent of the damaging rays.

6. A: Melanoma kills one person every hour in the United States, and its incidence has tripled among women in the last thirty years. Basal and squamous cell carcinomas are much more common than melanoma but also far less dangerous. All skin cancers are treatable when caught early.

7. B: I love these lotions because they mimic a natural tan without aging the skin or leaving it vulnerable to cancer. Unfortunately, the color they leave behind does *not* protect your skin from the sun. Some tanning lotions contain a sunscreen, which will give you at least some protection.

8. C: Benzophenone and avobenzone are chemical ingredients that absorb UV light before it can damage skin cells. Zinc oxide is a physical block that shields the skin from UV light the way that clothing does.

9. D: In other words, UV light is the reason for almost all forms of visible aging on the face. Just look at the inner part of your upper arm, which has probably been shielded from sunlight for most of your life, and you'll see what I mean.

10. A: Although prescription retinoids do an excellent job of repairing existing sun damage, they won't protect you from future injury. A moisturizer will only hydrate the skin. Applying topical antioxidants—and taking them orally—however, will give you added protection from UV light.

Leora's Story: Reducing Her SVA by Fifteen Years

You'd have to be living on a deserted island not to know that sun exposure is the number one reason your skin's virtual age is probably higher than you'd like it to be. More frightening still, it's the leading cause of skin cancer. Yet occasionally I meet someone who chooses to ignore this reality—even when it's written all over her face. When Leora, an Israeli-born patient, first came to see me, she was still in her twenties. She went to Florida as often as possible to soak up the sun, and when she wasn't outdoors in the sun, she was in a tanning salon evening out her color! It showed. Her eyes were perpetually puffy and inflamed, and although she was too young to have real wrinkles, her skin was so dark brown and leathery that it looked dirty.

In her throaty, hoarse voice (unfortunately, she was also a smoker), Leora asked me to laser away some of the large freckles that were taking over her face. I certainly had the equipment to do it, but I told her that it didn't make sense to start the process until she stopped tanning. Frankly, I'm not wild about the idea of using lasers and light sources on tanned skin—not

Myth Self-tanning lotions that give me a nice bronzy color protect my skin just as an actual tan does.

Truth Whereas a real tan does protect the skin from further sun damage, to some degree, your fake bronze color won't—not even one bit. Even if your lotion has an SPF 15 rating, it will guard against UV light only until you take your next shower. Furthermore, it is never applied thickly enough to really *be* an SPF 15, so make sure to wear a separate sunscreen as well.

only because it decreases the laser's effectiveness but, more important, because it dramatically increases the risk of treatment-induced pigment problems. I knew that I was dealing with a sun junkie, so I didn't push the issue. Instead, I discussed the ill effects of sun on the skin. Then I recommended that she gradually start using sunscreen and decrease the amount of time she spent baking outside. It took years for Leora to take my suggestions, but now, a decade and a half later, she has stopped smoking, wears sunscreen with regularity, and does her best to limit tanning. Would you believe that her SVA is significantly younger than it was the day she first walked into my office?

My patients, for the most part, are adults. I don't scold them or try to change their habits as if they're children, not even about something as serious as chronic tanning. For one thing, it's far more effective to give them the motivation to change on their own. (Realizing how unflattering leathery brown skin really is can be pretty convincing.) More to the point, no one likes to believe that he or she is going to have to give up sailing, tennis, golfing, gardening, and beach vacations for the rest of his or her life.

Dr. Dover Recommends

Drugstore

Chemical Sunscreens
- Skin Effects Active Continuous Spray Sunscreen SPF 45
- Skin Effects Sun Effects, with Dermaplex Technology SPF 30, 45, and 60 Lotion
- Skin Effects Sun Effects with Dermaplex Technology Active SPF 30 and 45
- Olay Complete Defense Daily Moisturizer SPF 30, Sensitive Skin
- Neutrogena Age Shield Sunblock with Helioplex, SPF 45
- Neutrogena Ultra Sheer Body Mist Sunblock SPF 45 with Helioplex
- Neutrogena Ultra Sheer Dry-Touch Sunblock with Helioplex, SPF 55 and SPF 70

- Aveeno Active Naturals Positively Radiant Daily Moisturizer with SPF 30 UVA/UVB Sunscreen
- Aveeno Active Naturals Positively Ageless Daily Moisturizer with SPF 30 UVA/UVB
- Aveeno Active Naturals Continuous Protection Sunblock Lotion with SPF 30, 45, and 55
- La Roche-Posay Anthelios 40 Sunscreen Cream, with Mexoryl SX

Physical Sunscreens
- Neutrogena Sensitive Skin Sunblock Lotion, SPF 30
- Burt's Bees Chemical-Free Sunscreen SPF 15
- Alba Botanica Fragrance Free Mineral Sunscreen SPF 18

Department Store and Doctor's Office

Chemical Sunscreens
- SkinCeuticals Active UV Defense SPF 15 UVA/UVB Protection with Mexoryl SX
- Murad Waterproof Sunblock SPF 30
- Sisley Broad Spectrum Sunscreen SPF 40, Colorless

Physical Sunscreens
- SkinCeuticals Physical UV Defense SPF 30
- DDF Organic Sunblock SPF 30

How the Sun Ages You

I enjoy my time in the sun, and I know that my much-loved outdoor activities keep me healthier in the long run than if I were spending hours on the couch in front of the TV. I know that the sun has some redeeming virtues, but I also know that Mae West's famous line "Too much of a good thing is . . . wonderful" doesn't apply to ultraviolet light. I wear sunscreen every day, and I use a double layer of it when I am enjoying outdoor activities. I never step onto a sailboat, a golf course, or a tennis court without a hat, and I do my best to avoid the bright midday sun, between the hours of 10 A.M. and 3 P.M. during the summer. After all this, I still wind up tanned, but if I didn't do these things, I'd be much darker and much more freckly and wrinkly.

Let's talk for a moment about exactly what ultraviolet light does to the skin and why it can cause your SVA to skyrocket like nothing else. There are two main types of UV light to worry about. The first, UVB, penetrates the skin and causes tanning, burning, and, eventually, skin cancer. The second, UVA, penetrates more deeply and causes more of the signs that we associate with maturing skin, like sallowness, wrinkling, and probably also some forms of skin cancer. UVA transmits right through window glass, which is why frequent drivers often have more sun damage on their hands and the left side of the face. Nearly all skin aging is related to sun exposure. In other words—and I really can't repeat this enough—a good sunscreen will keep you looking younger better than any fancy "age cream" sold at the department store.

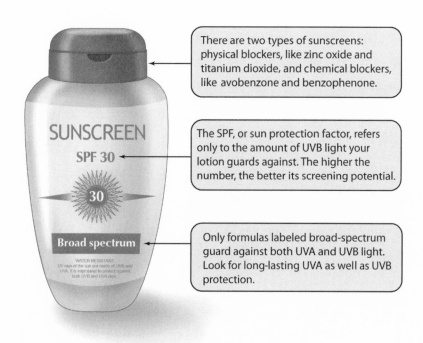

Choosing a sunscreen.

Myth Wearing an SPF 30 sunscreen means that I can stay in the sun thirty times longer than I could without any sunscreen.

Truth That SPF number is based on the assumption that you're slathering the lotion on liberally, which very few people do. In fact, studies show that the average person applies about one-fourth the amount of sunscreen that he or she should. Based on that calculation, when you put on an SPF 30, you'll get about sixteen times less protection than you think—probably something closer to an SPF 2. How does this relate to your next trip to the beach? Applied properly, an SPF 30 allows you to stay in the sun without burning thirty times longer than you would be able to without sunscreen. Applied the way most people use it, it allows you to stay in the sun only two times as long.

Recently I spoke with two construction workers who had figured out a way to apply sunscreen without making their hands too slippery to hold tools: they squirt it on their arms and then spread it on their face with their wrists. I never would have had that conversation ten years ago, and I'm thrilled that sun protection is turning into a national "religion." Nevertheless, many people still don't know how to choose a good sunscreen. Perhaps the following explanation will dispel any mystery for you once and for all.

The SPF, or sun protection factor, refers only to the amount of UVB light from which your lotion guards you. The higher the number, the better its screening potential. Although it used to be true that higher SPF formulas were typically thicker and less comfortable to wear, many of the most technologically advanced high-SPF formulas now contain incredibly fine particles of sunblocking ingredients, so they're more elegant and feel lighter than air on the skin. Generally, I advise patients to wear at least an SPF 15 when they're commuting to work and spending minimal time outside, then switch to an SPF 30 or higher when they will spend an extended amount of time outside. I also recommend that those who live in the northern United States and Canada upgrade to higher SPFs during the warm-weather months (April to October); those who live in the southern part of the country should wear higher SPFs year-round—at least an SPF 30, even when commuting to work. And make sure to reapply after every few hours of sun exposure.

Only formulas labeled "broad spectrum" guard against both UVA and UVB light. Parsol 1789 (or avobenzone), developed in the 1980s, was the first decent sunscreen to address UVA, but even that isn't perfect, since, ironically, it breaks down in sunlight. Recently, Neutrogena developed a UVA-shielding compound called Helioplex, Aveeno has created its Photobarrier Complex, and Skin Effects has developed Dermaplex. All these compounds stabilize avobenzone. The FDA recently approved L'Oreal's Mexoryl, a new sunscreening agent that delivers prolonged UVA protection. Not only do these products provide five hours of UVA sunscreen after one application, they also come in elegant light creams and lotions. They are not the pasty sunscreens that most people associate with high SPFs.

There are two types of sunscreens. (1) Physical blockers, like zinc oxide and titanium dioxide, do just what they say—they physically shield the skin from damaging rays, much like clothing does. Although these ingredients used to look white and chalky on the skin, the manufacturers have figured out how to micronize the particles so that they apply in an almost invisible film. (2) Chemical blocks, like avobenzone and benzophenone, absorb light before it can damage cells.

Myth Tanning beds are much safer than baking on the beach.

Truth There's no such thing as a healthy tanning bed; in fact, I believe they should all be banned—or, at the very least, much more aggressively regulated. Some salons claim that they filter out the burning spectrum called UVB. Even if that's true, you're getting plenty of damaging UVA rays. The truth is that if there's enough light in that box to tan you, there's enough to cause skin cancer and wrinkling. They go hand in hand.

Unfortunately, buying a good sunscreen doesn't mean that you're wearing nearly enough of it. I don't even want to *think* about how many people have tubes stashed in the bottom of their beach bags, or even under their bathroom sinks, but who rarely, if ever, get around to wearing the stuff. If you're truly diligent about applying it daily, my hat's off to you. Just keep in mind that even the best-intentioned among us probably aren't applying quite enough of it.

Exactly how much sunscreen should you put on each day to knock down your skin's virtual age several notches and keep it there? It depends on what your plans are and how much skin you're exposing. I usually say that it takes about one ounce (or a full shot glass) of sunscreen to cover your entire body. One thing I know for sure: if at the end of the summer you're still squirting from the same tube that you bought before Memorial Day weekend, you need an education in application. Studies show that an SPF 30 sunscreen, applied in the quantities most people use, yields an SPF of only 2! Ideally, you should coat every exposed patch of skin with a thick layer of sunscreen, and continue to reapply it every few hours you remain outside. (Apply more often after sweating or swimming.)

Remember that even the best-made, best-applied formula screens out only 98 percent of those damaging rays. This means that 2 percent of those rays are hitting any exposed skin—and increasing your SVA— every minute you're outside. The best way to limit sun damage is to steer clear of sun exposure by using protective clothing and practicing sun avoidance. Walk on the shady side of the street and stand under trees and outdoor shelters as much as possible. Look for sun hats with a brim of at least seven centimeters (roughly the distance from your thumb to your index finger when they are spread apart). Keep in mind that the average T-shirt offers protection equivalent to only an SPF 6 to 10. I vividly remember going to Crane's Beach in Massachusetts about fifteen years ago with my wife, Tania (who is also a dermatologist), my friend who was the director of skin cancer awareness in Canada, and his wife. It was a gorgeous summer day: sunny and in the high 80s. We were covered head to toe in sweatpants, long-sleeve shirts, huge broad-brimmed hats, and big sunglasses. We looked like aliens, but we were the only ones there who weren't tanning (and likely burning) like mad. Everyone else on the beach was wearing skimpy bathing suits and probably just enough sunscreen to keep them from becoming as red as a lobster.

There are now clothing lines that are specifically designated as sun-protective—clothes that look breezy, lightweight, and really attractive. My favorite places to find them are www.solumbra.com and www.coolibar.com, but you can also buy them in stores that sell outdoor and sporting clothes. Don't forget that wearing sunscreen and night lotions—along with creams containing antioxidants, retinoids, and other anti-aging ingredients—will help to repair existing UV damage, turning back the clock on your skin's virtual age. (For a list of my favorite antioxidants, see page 65.)

Dr. Dover Recommends

Drugstore

Sunscreens with Antioxidants
- Skin Effects Sun Effects Line
- Neutrogena Anti-Oxidant Age Reverse Day Lotion SPF 20
- Eucerin Q10 Anti-Wrinkle Sensitive Skin Crème and Lotion SPF 15
- La Roche-Posay Biomedic Facial Shield SPF 20
- Coppertone Ultrasheer Faces SPF 30

Wrinkle-Smoothing Sunscreens
- Skin Effects Daily Anti-Aging Treatment Cream SPF 15
- Skin Effects Lightweight Moisturizing Soufflé SPF 30+
- Olay Regenerist UV Defense Regenerating Lotion
- Olay Anti-Wrinkle Daily SPF 15 Lotion
- Neutrogena Healthy Skin Anti-Wrinkle Intensive Deep Wrinkle Moisturizing Treatment SPF 20
- Aveeno Active Naturals Positively Ageless Daily Moisturizer SPF 30 UVA/UVB
- RoC Anti-Wrinkle Retinol Actif Pur Day SPF 15
- Vichy LiftActiv PRO Pro-Fibre Anti-Wrinkle and Firming Care SPF 15

Myth Tanning will clear up my acne.

Truth This is somewhat true. A large, well-done study in the 1970s showed that ultraviolet light didn't really make acne improve. So for years, I told my patients that the reason tanning seems to make acne look better was that it simply hid the pimples. Also, people tend to tan in the summer, when they're under less stress, and when you reduce stress, acne usually gets better. Now it turns out that UV and visible light *can* actually help to clear pimples. However—and this is a *big* however—the ill effects of tanning are far worse than the beneficial effect of the light on blemishes. On the positive side, there's a slew of safe, non-UV light treatments for acne. They're not perfect, but they're getting better every year.

Sunscreen Moisturizers

- Skin Effects Lightweight Moisturizing Soufflé SPF 30+
- Skin Effects Daily Anti-Aging Body Lotion SPF 30+
- Olay Definity Deep Penetrating Foaming UV Moisturizer, SPF 15, Fragrance Free
- Olay Complete Plus Ultra-Rich Day Cream SPF 15
- Neutrogena Healthy Skin Visibly Even Daily SPF 15 Moisturizer
- Aveeno Active Naturals Ultra-Calming Daily Moisturizer with UVA/UVB Sunscreen
- RoC Age Diminishing Daily Moisturizer SPF 15
- Cetaphil Daily Facial Moisturizer SPF 15 with Parsol 1789
- Eucerin Protective Moisture Lotion SPF 30
- La Roche-Posay Biomedic Gentle Moisturizing Lotion SPF 15
- Vichy Nutrilogie 1 Intensive Nourishing Moisturizer Lotion
- Purpose Dual Treatment Moisture Lotion with SPF 15

Self-Tanning Sunscreens

- Skin Effects Daily Self-Tanning Moisturizer SPF 15
- Jergens Natural Glow Face Daily Moisturizer SPF 20

- Olay Touch of Sun Daily UV Facial Moisturizer Lighter/Medium
- Neutrogena Summer Glow Daily Moisturizer SPF 20
- Coppertone Oil Free Sunless Tanning Lotion

Department Store and Doctor's Office

Sunscreens with Antioxidants

- SkinCare Prescription Day Anti-Aging Moisturizer AHA with SPF 15
- Dr. Brandt Daily UV Protection SPF 30 Colorless
- DDF Matte Finish Photo-Age Protection SPF 30
- Murad Oil-Free Sunblock SPF 30
- Orlane Anti-Wrinkle Sun Serum for the Face

Wrinkle-Smoothing Sunscreens

- SkinCare Prescription Day Anti-Aging Moisturizer AHA with SPF 15
- SkinMedica TNS Ultimate Daily Moisturizer + SPF 20
- Murad Perfecting Day Cream SPF 30
- Patricia Wexler M.D. Dermatology Universal Anti-Aging Moisturizer SPF 30
- La Prairie Anti-Aging Emulsion SPF 30
- Orlane Anti-Aging Sun Cream SPF 30

Addicted to Sunlight and Tanning?

I wasn't joking when I referred to Leora as a sun junkie. A recent study shows that UV light stimulates the same opioid receptors in the body that some addictive drugs, like morphine and heroin, do. I'm telling you this because I want you to stop and think the next time you feel inexplicably drawn to the tanning salon or to that patch of unshaded sand on the beach. Understanding *why* sun exposure makes you feel so good, especially if you've been basking in it all your life, is the first step to curbing your UV addiction. Trust me, your skin will thank you for it.

Sunscreen Moisturizers
- SkinMedica TNS Ultimate Daily Moisturizer + SPF 20
- SkinCeuticals Ultimate UV Defense SPF 30 Moisturizing Broad-Spectrum UVA/UVB Sunscreen
- DDF Daily Protective Moisturizer SPF 15
- Kinerase Cream with SPF 30
- Murad Redness Therapy Correcting Moisturizer SPF 15
- Patricia Wexler M.D. Dermatology Acnescription Oil-Free Hydrator SPF 30 for Acne
- Clé de Peau Protective Moisturizer

Self-Tanning Sunscreens
- Kiehl's Sunscreen Crème SPF 15
- Dr. Brandt Daily UV Protection SPF 30 Face, in light bronze or medium bronze
- Murad Oil-Free Sunblock Sheer Tint SPF 15
- Sisley Broad Spectrum Sunscreen SPF 25 Amber
- Orlane Anti-Wrinkle Self-Tanner SPF 8

Grace's Story: Catching Skin Cancer Early

Grace, a program administrator and the mother of two beautiful children, was forty-two years old but had an SVA of nearly fifty when she first asked me about the scattered brown spots and crow's feet marring her complexion, the increasing redness on her cheeks, and the very early-stage sagging that had just begun to weigh down the sides of her face. She was a busy woman, and she wanted quick answers, but before I could begin to address her cosmetic issues, I had to determine what was causing the red scaly patch over her right eyebrow. When I asked her about it, she admitted that the patch had been there for at least a year but said she wasn't worried about it. I was.

I immediately told her that I was concerned that this could be skin cancer and that we had to take a biopsy of the spot before we did anything else. The results revealed that Grace's spot was indeed a squamous cell carcinoma, an increasingly common form of skin cancer that, fortunately, is easily treatable when detected early. (If it's caught too late, the growths can leave disfiguring scars or, much worse, slowly invade other parts of the body.) Grace was one of the lucky ones: we found her patch early. In the past fourteen months, we've treated it with three different topical anticancer creams. Just recently, she returned to me for a follow-up exam, and to our delight, the biopsy revealed that the spot has cleared completely. At last we can begin to tackle the crow's feet and brown spots.

This book is about reducing your skin's virtual age, which will certainly make you look much better. It will also make your complexion *healthier* by reducing your risk of skin cancer. Skin cancer is the most common form of cancer, and in the past thirty years its incidence has tripled in women under age forty. Melanoma, the deadliest form of all, kills one person every hour.

On the upside, I remind my patients that the disease is among the most curable of all cancers when diagnosed early. Early detection leads to a cure in more than 99 percent of all melanomas. Everyone should have his or her primary care physician check the skin during each annual physical. Any suspicious skin spots should be checked by a dermatologist. If you are particularly at risk (that is, if you have a family history of any kind of skin cancer, have already had a skin cancer, or have light eyes and/or fair skin), I recommend that you have your skin checked by a dermatologist on a regular basis. I also tell all my patients to scan their own bodies every month; for women, this is ideally just before or after their monthly breast self-exam. Women are particularly good at finding their own skin cancer and that of their partners. Nothing beats a monthly self-exam to identify a skin cancer early.

Basal cell cancers can look as innocent as a skin-colored mole or a pimple that just won't clear up. Squamous cell cancers can be found in a pink scaly or crusty patch of skin. Melanoma begins in an existing mole that has changed in color, shape, or size, or it can emerge out of nowhere, as a brown, black, or pink mark that looks flat or slightly raised. Moles that exhibit one or more of the following "ABCDE" qualities should be checked by a dermatologist, because they might be a melanoma:

(A) Asymmetry

(B) An uneven or scalloped border

(C) A variety of color shades

(D) A diameter that's larger than a pencil eraser

(E) A shape, size, color, or elevation that is evolving or changing; sudden bleeding or itching is also suspicious

Although topical cream treatments are being developed for basal cell and squamous cell cancer, the treatment of choice for most early skin cancers and all melanomas is surgical removal. Early treatment of all three types of skin cancers leads to a cure, so early detection is crucial.

The Game Plan: Six Do-at-Home Steps for Lowering Your SVA

1. Pile on the sunscreen. Since it helps to shield your skin from aging UV rays, sunscreen is the most effective wrinkle cream you'll ever buy. Applying it to all exposed areas should be as much a part of your morning routine as brushing your teeth.

2. Then pile on more. I'll say this again, because it bears repeating: studies show that an SPF 30 sunscreen applied in the quantities that most people use yields an SPF of only 2. That's why I apply at least two coats at first, then reapply for every few hours I remain outside, and even more often after sweating or swimming.

3. Don't forget your hands. I often notice that my patients' hands look much older—and have a higher SVA—than the rest of their skin, especially the face. That's because even though our hands are possibly the most exposed parts of us, no one thinks to protect them. Regardless of the season, coat the backs of your hands with sunscreen daily, and don't forget to reapply after each time you wash your hands. It might be a good idea to replace your ordinary hand cream with a rich sunscreen moisturizer.

4. Read the label. All sunscreens are not created equal. Look for a formula labeled "broad spectrum," meaning that it will protect you from both UVA and UVB forms of light. Aim for an SPF of at least 15, and higher if you're planning on spending an extended amount of time outside or if you live in the South. Keep in mind that this number refers only to its ability to shield you from UVB rays, at least for now. You can read more about how to decode a sunscreen label on page 102.

5. Buy extra skin-protection insurance. Even the best, most expertly applied sunscreen can do only so much to block the sun's damaging rays. Compensate by wearing hats and other sun-protective clothing. Be sure that at least one of your treatment products contains antioxidants, then load up your diet with antioxidant vitamins and food filled with antioxidants, like berries, tomatoes, and green tea.

6. Check your skin. Having a low SVA means more than simply having beautiful skin; it means having *healthy* skin as well. Even if you're not a sun worshiper, scan your body often for suspicious-looking moles and spots. Have your primary care doctor or dermatologist perform a skin check at least once a year. For more on how to separate suspicious spots from benign ones, see pages 110–111.

the prescription

Until recently, it seemed unthinkable that anyone could actually knock years off his or her appearance *without* having a blepharoplasty (eyelid surgery), a brow lift, or a face-lift. Although there's nothing wrong with turning to the scalpel, these surgical procedures come with certain risks, significant recovery time, and a substantial price tag. In the previous section I discussed the growing world of topical treatments—the serums, lotions, and creams you can buy at the local drugstore or department store—and their incredible ability to turn back the clock. I've seen amazing things happen to patients who find the right combination of these products and who have the discipline to use them day after day; honestly, I've even been astounded by their progress. Your skin can astound you, too, as long as you find *your* SVA-lowering youth equation.

6

No Surgery, No Kidding
Dr. Dover's Six-Week Plan for Younger-Looking Skin

If you've read everything up to this point, you have a very good idea of what topicals are available and how they work. Now I want to give you the key to unlocking a more youthful appearance for your complexion; I want to offer you a six-week prescription for younger-looking, younger-*behaving* skin. Here's how this chapter works: On the pages that follow, I've included six regimens for skin by age decade, ranging from twentysomething to seventysomething and beyond, along with short stories of patients who put these regimens into action. Each decade's section reflects your SVA: your skin's *virtual* age, not its actual age. Based on your results from the quiz you took in chapter 1, find the section that reflects your SVA and follow the protocol as closely as you can. You'll see that I've offered two or three product recommendations for each step, except for the sections that suggest prescription creams or in-office treatments. These recommendations are based on the assumption that you have fairly normal skin—not excessively dry, oily, or sensitive skin. For a more complete list of my favorite products for all skin types, along with more information about the ingredients I'm suggesting, refer back to the appropriate section: chapter 3, "Cleanse"; chapter 4, "Treat"; or chapter 5, "Prevent."

If you follow my suggested prescription dutifully every morning and every night, you *will* see a marked change in your complexion within six weeks—and even more improvement over time. You will see brighter skin, a decrease in uneven pigmentation and fine lines, and eventually you will enjoy a firmer, healthier-looking face. For each decade, I've offered basic morning and evening recommendations for cleansing, treating, and preventing damage, along with "extra credit" options you can add if you have time. (You'll notice that each decade's prescription builds on the one before it.) If you're truly ambitious and want to maximize your skin's response, you might even skip ahead and incorporate a product or two from a later decade. For example, even though I start prescribing retinoids for women with an SVA of thirtysomething, there's nothing to stop you from starting to use them in your twenties.

My only caveat is that certain skin types improve more quickly than others. Those who have good skin texture, but whose skin looks tired and dull and might have some sun-induced brown spots, will see the most rapid improvement. In six weeks, dull skin will look much brighter, and brown spots will fade to some extent, at least. You might have an older SVA with a great deal of accumulated sun damage when you start my plan, but if your major issue is tired, dull skin, you will still see significant improvement in tone, color, and radiance.

If, however, the biggest problem with your skin is sagging and loss of skin tone, and you have significant sun damage, you can expect to see less improvement during the first six weeks. That's because it will simply take longer to undo all of the injury of the past. In this case, you'll have to be more patient—and, ideally, put as many potent ingredients into your regimen as possible. Be assured, however, that after six weeks, your skin will look brighter, healthier, and younger. Are you ready to begin?

A Skin-Care Regimen for Your SVA: Twenties

What you see in the mirror: a radiant glow with very few (if any) fine lines that appear only when you smile or frown. You might have a handful of brown spots, which is an early sign of past sun damage. You might also have some acne, either a residual case or a frustrating new one.

Cleanse

Morning and night. Wash with your favorite cleanser(s); see page 41 for more on specific types of cleansers based on your skin's needs. If you're battling acne, consider a formula that contains salicylic acid or benzoyl peroxide. Just be careful not to overuse medicated formulas, because they can lead to irritation.

Dr. Dover Recommends

Drugstore

- Skin Effects Gentle Foaming Cleanser
- Neutrogena One Step Gentle Cleanser
- Aveeno Active Naturals Clear Complexion Foaming Cleanser

Department Store and Doctor's Office

- SkinCare Prescription System Cleanser
- SkinCeuticals Foaming Cleanser

Extra credit: night. Once or twice a week, polish the skin with either an exfoliating cleanser that contains round soft grains or a chemical exfoliant like alpha hydroxy acid or fruit enzymes. Since these formulas remove the uppermost layer of dead skin cells, thus increasing the penetration of whatever cream or lotion you apply after, it's best to use them at night before moving on to the "treat" step.

Dr. Dover Recommends

Drugstore

- Skin Effects Deep Cleaning Enzyme Scrub
- Olay Smooth Skin Exfoliating Scrub with Gentle Microbeads
- Neutrogena Healthy Skin Visibly Even Foaming Cleanser

Department Store and Doctor's Office

- SkinCare Prescription Exfoliator
- Sisley Botanical Buff & Wash Facial Gel

Treat

Night. After cleansing the skin, apply a lotion, cream, or serum that contains anti-aging ingredients (like glycolic acid, vitamin A derivatives like retinol, vitamin C, green tea, or coenzyme Q10) to help brighten the skin and slowly smooth away emerging lines and brown spots.

Dr. Dover Recommends

Drugstore

- Skin Effects Resurfacing Effects Skin Renewal System
- La Roche-Posay Biomedic Retinol 15
- Neutrogena Anti-Oxidant Age Reverse Night Cream

Department Store and Doctor's Office

- SkinCare Prescription Night Anti-Aging Moisturizer with Retinol
- SkinCeuticals C + AHA
- Murad Essential-C Daily Renewal Complex

If acne is a problem, add over-the-counter products that contain benzoyl peroxide or salicylic acid, or talk to your dermatologist about prescription treatments that might be right for you.

Dr. Dover Recommends

Drugstore

- Skin Effects Acne Treatment System
- Olay Total Effects 7-in-1 Anti-Aging Moisturizer Plus Blemish Control
- Neutrogena Complete Acne Therapy System

Department Store and Doctor's Office

- NeoStrata Blemish Treatment Gel
- Rodan + Fields Unblemish
- Patricia Wexler M.D. Dermatology Anti-Acne Starter Kit

Extra credit: morning. If you're going to dab on a moisturizer anyway, why not choose a formula with anti-aging capabilities? (As I said earlier, I believe that no one should let a twelve-hour period go by without doing *something* to turn back the clock.) Some of my favorite moisturizers contain hydrating ingredients, like hyaluronic acid and glycerin; antioxidants, like vitamin C, green tea, idebenone, or coenzyme Q10; and anti-aging ingredients, like glycolic acid, vitamin A derivatives, vitamins C and E, alpha lipoic acid, and peptides. The antioxidants will help to mop up the damaging free radicals that the skin has generated in response to sun exposure, pollutants, and other environmental factors.

Dr. Dover Recommends

Drugstore

- Skin Effects Daily Anti-Aging Treatment Cream SPF 15
- Aveeno Active Naturals Clear Complexion Daily Moisturizer
- Vichy Normaderm Anti-Imperfection Hydrating Care

Department Store and Doctor's Office

- SkinCare Prescription Day Anti-Aging Moisturizer AHA with SPF 15

- DDF Retinol Energizing Moisturizer
- Dr. Brandt Liquid Synergy

Night. To stave off emerging fine lines, ask your doctor to pre-scribe a retinoid cream. You might start by rubbing it on every other night, until your skin is used to it, and eventually work up to using it every night. If you are concerned about the irritation and wish to skip the doctor's office visit, try Skin Effects Cell 2 Cell Continuous Action Anti-Wrinkle Care.

Prevent

Morning. If you're going to be outside for much of the day, apply a good-quality, broad-spectrum sunscreen (one that shields your skin from both UVA and UVB rays) to *all* the areas that will be exposed to the sun, then reapply every few hours you remain outside. For infor-mation on the various types of sunscreens available and on how to choose the best one for you, see pages 103–106. Keep in mind that it takes about one ounce (or a full shot glass) of the stuff to cover your entire body. Studies show that an SPF 30 sunscreen, applied in the quantities that most people use, yields an SPF of only about 2. During the week, or on days when your outdoor activities are limited, you should use a combination product that contains a sunscreen and anti-aging ingredients. Reapplication on these days is less important.

Dr. Dover Recommends

Drugstore
- Skin Effects Sun Effects Active SPF 45
- Aveeno Active Naturals Continuous Protection Sunblock Lotion for the Face with SPF 30

Department Store and Doctor's Office
- Patricia Wexler M.D. Dermatology Acnescription Oil-Free Hydrator SPF 30 for Acne
- Murad Oil-Free Sunblock Sheer Tint SPF 15

Hannah's Story: Starting Her Routine Early

At age twenty-six, Hannah had never been to a dermatologist before. This is hardly surprising: except for an occasional pimple, she had a relatively problem-free complexion. It was only after admiring her best friend's clear, radiant skin one night that she began to think about seeing a professional. Hannah's friend gave her my card and suggested that she book an appointment.

When she walked in, I asked her the same question that I ask all my patients: What bothers you most about your skin? Hannah couldn't name anything specific at first. She pointed vaguely to the cluster of small pimples on her forehead and to the large pores on and around her nose. "I don't know," she finally said. "I was looking at pictures of myself from just a couple of years ago. It's not that I look old, but all of a sudden my face doesn't seem to have the same glow."

Even without seeing those old photographs, I could understand what Hannah meant. When I took a close look, it was clear that the very early signs of sun damage had begun to emerge on her face in the form of small, almost imperceptible blotches and the faintest fine lines around her eyes. Perhaps most noticeable was that her overall skin tone did look a bit dull. When I asked Hannah what she used on her face, she shrugged and answered, "Usually whatever bar of soap is in the shower and maybe a moisturizer in the winter." Bingo.

Since she was still a few years away from her thirties. with a complexion that usually "behaved" itself, Hannah assumed that she could just leave it alone. She wasn't the type of person to spend much time in front of the mirror grooming morning or night. The short, simple list of products that I put together with her was very affordable, available at any drugstore, and extremely effective. Best of all, for her, they were very easy and speedy to use. I suggested that Hannah save the bar soap for her body and treat her face morning and night to a gentle foaming wash—one that smells great and leaves her skin feeling soft, not tight. Since her skin showed no signs of sensitivity, I gave her a sample of a fruit enzyme exfoliating scrub to use a few times a week to restore her complexion's luster. I suggested that every morning she apply a mild benzoyl peroxide cream to her entire face (not just to the acne-prone areas), followed by a sunscreen that contains moisturizer with anti-aging ingredients. For "extra credit," she could use a sunscreen with a brightening agent like hydroquinone, kojic acid, soy, Sepiwhite MSH, or green or black tea. At night, I suggested, she should use an additional lotion that contains brightening face cream. To prevent further sun damage later, I told her, she should not leave her house without applying a broad-spectrum sunblock on all exposed skin.

By the time Hannah came in for her follow-up appointment six weeks later, I noticed a marked improvement in her skin. More important, so did she. "Honestly, I think my skin looks cleaner and less dull than it did in those old photos," she said, "and I haven't seen a zit in two weeks." In just a few weeks Hannah had become a believer. Now try telling her that skin care doesn't matter.

A Skin-Care Regimen for Your SVA: Thirties

What you see in the mirror: fairly smooth skin that still bounces back when you pinch it. Your natural glow has likely begun to fade, thanks to slowing cell turnover, and fine lines might be appearing around your eyes and forehead. At the same time, brown spots are accumulating, especially along the sides of your face, and tiny red veins might be cropping up around your nose and on your cheeks.

Cleanse

Morning and night. Wash with your favorite cleanser (see page 41 for information on specific types). If you're still battling acne, consider a formula that contains salicylic acid or benzoyl peroxide. Just be careful not to overuse medicated formulas, because they can lead to irritation.

Dr. Dover Recommends

Drugstore

- Skin Effects Gentle Foaming Cleanser
- Cetaphil Daily Facial Cleanser for Normal to Oily Skin
- L'Oreal Ideal Balance Foaming Cream Cleanser
- Olay Regenerist Daily Regenerating Cleanser

Department Store and Doctor's Office

- SkinCare Prescription Cleanser
- La Prairie Cellular Comforting Cleansing Emulsion
- SkinCeuticals Simply Clean

Extra credit: night. A few times a week, polish the skin with either an exfoliating cleanser that contains round soft grains or a chemical exfoliant like alpha hydroxy acid or fruit enzymes. These formulas remove the uppermost layer of dead skin cells, which is especially helpful now because your cell turnover is slowing down. Furthermore, exfoliating increases the penetration of whatever cream or lotion you apply immediately after, so it's best to exfoliate at night before moving on to the "treat" step.

Dr. Dover Recommends

Drugstore

- Skin Effects Deep Cleaning Enzyme Scrub
- Olay Definity Pore Refining Scrub
- Pond's Dramatic Results Age-Defying Cleansing Towelettes with Vitamin A, Retinol, and Collagen

Department Store and Doctor's Office

- SkinMedica Skin Polisher
- RéVive Cleanser Exfoliante

Treat

Morning. Start with a skin-brightening product that contains an ingredient like hydroquinone, kojic acid, arbutin, soy, Sepiwhite MSH, or green or black tea to combat your sun-induced brown spots and to help brighten your skin.

Dr. Dover Recommends

Drugstore

- Skin Effects Advanced Brightening Complex
- Aveeno Active Naturals Positively Radiant Eye Brightening Cream

Department Store and Doctor's Office

- Révive Blanche Whiten, Lighten, Brighten
- Dr. Brandt Laser Lightening Day Lotion
- DDF Intensive Holistic Lightener

Apply a moisturizer with anti-aging ingredients. (If you choose one with sunscreen, that's even better.) Some of my favorite moisturizers contain hydrating ingredients, like hyaluronic acid and glycerin; anti-aging ingredients, like glycolic acid, peptides, and vitamins A (retinol, retinyl palmitate), C (ascorbic acid, ascorbyl palmitate), and E (tocopheryl); and antioxidants, like vitamin C, green tea, coenzyme Q10, and idebenone. This will help to mop up damaging free radicals that the skin has generated in response to sun exposure, pollutants, and other environmental factors.

Dr. Dover Recommends

Drugstore

- Skin Effects Lightweight Moisturizing Soufflé SPF 30
- Olay Definity Penetrating Foaming Moisturizer

Department Store and Doctor's Office

- SkinMedica TNS Ultimate Daily Moisturizer + SPF 20
- Orlane Anti-Wrinkle After-Sun Balm for the Face SPF 15

Night. Ask your dermatologist to prescribe a retinoid cream to speed up your sluggish cell turnover, increase collagen production, and help the skin to look and feel younger. Depending on which retinoid you use, you might notice that your complexion feels drier, especially during the first few weeks of use. Be sure to apply it when your face is completely dry, then apply a night moisturizer a few minutes after putting on your retinoid (see pages 59–63 for information on retinoids). If you're prone to facial flushing, consider an over-the-counter gel or lotion that reduces redness.

Extra credit: morning and night. Apply an eye cream that contains rich moisturizers, like glycerin, cyclopentasiloxane, silicone, and dimethicone, as well as brighteners, like vitamin C derivatives, licorice extract (glycerrhetinic acid), and hydroquinone. If fine lines surrounding the eyes are a problem, be sure that your cream contains vitamin A. If you're suffering from puffiness around the eyes, look for a cream with caffeine, alpha lipoic acid, or peptides. Apply the eye cream at night as well.

Dr. Dover Recommends

Drugstore

- Skin Effects Dual Action Under Eye Therapy
- Olay Regenerist Eye Lifting Serum
- Neutrogena Age Reverse Eye Cream

Department Store and Doctor's Office

- Patricia Wexler M.D. Dermatology Under-Eye Brightening Cream
- Murad Lighten and Brighten Eye Treatment

Anytime. Occasionally, book a series of light glycolic acid peels, microdermabrasion, or a vibraderm treatment. Performed in a dermatologist's office or in a doctor-supervised medical spa, these procedures will encourage deeper cell turnover, cause brown spots to fade, and smooth fine lines, but mostly they will help to polish and brighten your skin.

Prevent

Morning. Ideally, your moisturizer contains sunscreen. However, if it doesn't, or if you're going to be outside for much of the day, apply a good-quality, broad-spectrum sunscreen (one that shields you from both UVA and UVB rays) to *all* areas of the skin that will be exposed to the sun. Then reapply it every few hours that you remain outside. (See pages 103–106 for more information on sunscreens.) Keep in mind that it takes about one ounce (or a full shot glass) of the stuff to cover your entire body. Studies show that an SPF 30 sunscreen, applied in the quantities that most people use, yields an SPF of only about 2. During the week, or on days when your outdoor activities are limited, you should use a combination product that contains a sunscreen and anti-aging ingredients. Reapplication on these days is less important.

Dr. Dover Recommends

Drugstore

- Skin Effects Sun Effects Active SPF 45
- Neutrogena Ultra Sheer Dry-Touch Sunblock with Helioplex SPF 55

Department Store and Doctor's Office

- SkinCeuticals Active UV Defense SPF 15 UVA/UVB protection with Mexoryl SX
- DDF Daily Matte SPF 15

Josie's Story: The Former Lifeguard

As a teenager, Josie had spent her summers working as a lifeguard at the beach and surfing on her days off. Moreover, the thirty-five-year-old admitted to me on her first visit, she hadn't always been diligent about protecting her skin from the sun. So even though she was frustrated to see brown spots appearing on her outer cheeks, she wasn't shocked.

"I know I'm paying for my past," she said to me. She assured me that she was diligent about sun protection now, but she knew that this would do nothing for the UV damage she had already accumulated.

Josie had friends who had lasered off their brown spots, but she just wasn't ready to do that yet. She was thrilled when I told her that we could make a lot of headway with the right topical regimen. Although the glycolic cream she was using was a great way to brighten her skin and lighten her brown spots, it just wasn't strong enough for her purposes, so I upgraded her to a 4 percent hydroquinone cream to fade her blotches and brighten her skin more quickly. For the evening, I prescribed a retinoid to improve the overall quality of her skin, specifically to brighten and smooth her complexion but also to help the hydroquinone lighten the sun-induced spots. Meanwhile, I told her, it wouldn't hurt to book a series of six light glycolic acid peels once every week or two to gently lift away more of that past sun damage and reveal younger-looking skin underneath. I also asked Josie to switch her basic moisturizer—which really wasn't doing anything for her skin—for one with anti-aging and antioxidant ingredients.

Josie was skeptical—and, I'll admit, even I didn't know how well or how quickly this new set of products would go to work on her brown spots. Thus I was overjoyed to find that her skin looked much better and that the brown spots had faded considerably after six weeks—and significantly after six months. Josie is still considering laser treatments in the future, particularly for her increasingly blotchy arms and hands. For now, however, she's dutifully slathering on her brightening topicals and an extra layer of sunscreen.

A Skin-Care Regimen for Your SVA: Forties

What you see in the mirror: more dullness, especially in sun-damaged spots, along with a growing number of brown spots, fine lines, and deepening creases. Because of a gradual fat loss in your cheeks and an increasing skin laxity, your skin isn't quite as taut as it used to be.

Cleanse

Morning and night. Wash with your favorite cleanser. If your skin is beginning to feel more dry than usual, consider switching to a creamier formula (see page 41 for specific types of cleansers).

Dr. Dover Recommends

Drugstore

- Skin Effects Redness Control Calming Gel Cleanser
- Olay Regenerist Daily Regenerating Cleanser
- Vichy Calming Cleansing Solution

Department Store and Doctor's Office

- SkinMedica Facial Cleanser
- N.V. Perricone M.D. Olive Oil Polyphenols Gentle Cleanser

Extra credit: night. Once or twice a week, polish the skin with either an exfoliating cleanser that contains round soft grains or a chemical exfoliant like alpha hydroxy acid or fruit enzymes. These formulas remove the uppermost layer of dead skin cells, which is especially helpful now, as your cell turnover continues to slow down. Because exfoliating increases the penetration of whatever cream or lotion you apply immediately after, it's best to exfoliate at night before moving on to the "treat" step.

Dr. Dover Recommends

Drugstore

- Skin Effects Deep Cleaning Enzyme Scrub
- RoC Daily Microdermabrasion Cleansing Disks
- Aveeno Skin Brightening Daily Scrub
- La Roche-Posay Biomedic LHA Cleansing Gel

Department Store and Doctor's Office

- SkinCeuticals Cleansing Cream
- Dr. Brandt Microdermabrasion

Treat

Morning. Start with a skin-brightening product that contains an ingredient like hydroquinone, kojic acid, soy, Sepiwhite MSH, or green or black tea to combat your sun-induced brown spots and to help brighten your skin.

Dr. Dover Recommends

Drugstore

- Skin Effects Advanced Brightening Complex
- Olay Definity Illuminating Eye Cream
- L'Oreal Dermo-Expertise Age Perfect Double Action De-Crinkling & Illuminating Treatment

Department Store and Doctor's Office

- Kinerase Brightening Anti-Aging System
- La Prairie The Radiance Collection
- La Mer The Radiant Facial

Apply a moisturizer that will also work on wrinkles and dulling skin; it's even better if it contains sunscreen. Some of my favorites have hydrating ingredients, like hyaluronic acid and glycerin; anti-aging ingredients, like glycolic acid, peptides, and vitamins A (retinol, retinyl palmitate), C (ascorbic acid, ascorbyl palmitate), and E (tocopheryl); and antioxidants, like vitamin C, green tea, coenzyme Q10, or idebenone. The antioxidants will help to mop up damaging free radicals that the skin has generated in response to sun exposure, pollutants, and other environmental factors.

Dr. Dover Recommends

Drugstore

- Skin Effects Cell 2 Cell Continuous Action Anti-Wrinkle Care
- Olay Total Effects 7-in-1 Anti-Aging Moisturizer
- Olay Regenerist Daily Regenerating Serum

Department Store and Doctor's Office
- SkinMedica TNS Ultimate Daily Moisturizer + SPF 20
- Prevage Anti-Aging Treatment

Night. If you haven't done so already, ask your dermatologist to prescribe a retinoid cream to speed sluggish cell turnover, increase collagen production, and help the skin to look and feel younger. Depending on which retinoid you use, you might notice that your complexion feels drier, especially during the first few weeks of use. Applying a night moisturizer five minutes after putting on your retinoid will help. (See pages 59–63 for information on retinoids.)

After putting on the prescription retinoid, lightly coat both the face and the neck with a skin-firming product. Look for formulas with tightening ingredients like GABA, lycopene, DMAE, and alpha lipoic acid.

Dr. Dover Recommends

Drugstore
- Skin Effects Firming Face and Neck Cream
- Olay Night of Olay Firming Cream

Department Store and Doctor's Office
- N.V. Perricone M.D. Neuropeptide Firming Moisturizer
- Dr. Brandt Laser in a Bottle

Apply an eye cream that contains rich moisturizers, like glycerin, cyclopentasiloxane, silicone, and dimethicone, as well as brighteners, like vitamin C derivatives and licorice extract (glycerrhetinic acid). If fine lines surrounding the eyes are a problem, be sure that your cream has vitamin A. If you're suffering from puffiness around the eyes, look for a cream with caffeine and alpha lipoic acid.

Dr. Dover Recommends

Drugstore
- Skin Effects Intensive Eye Treatment or Dual Action Under Eye Therapy

- Neutrogena Visibly Firm Eye Cream
- Aveeno Active Naturals Positively Ageless Eye Serum

Department Store and Doctor's Office

- SkinCare Prescription Anti-Aging Eye Cream
- Prevage Eye Anti-Aging Moisturizing Treatment
- Dr. Brandt Lineless Eye Cream
- SkinCeuticals Eye Gel AOX+

Extra credit: night. If your skin is starting to feel more parched than usual, adding a heavier night cream—a moisturizer that's slightly richer than daytime formulas and, of course, doesn't have sunscreen—will make your complexion look more plump and dewy when you wake up. There's no reason not to choose a formula that contains anti-aging components.

Dr. Dover Recommends

Drugstore

- Skin Effects Intensive Overnight Repair Cream
- Neutrogena Light Night Cream
- Olay Regenerist Deep Hydration Regenerating Cream

Department Store and Doctor's Office

- SkinCare Prescription Night Anti-Aging Moisturizer with Retinol
- RéVive Moisturizing Renewal Cream

Anytime. Occasionally, book a series of light glycolic acid peels, microdermabrasion, or a vibraderm treatment. Performed in a dermatologist's office or in a doctor-supervised medical spa, these procedures encourage deeper cell turnover, cause brown spots to fade, and smooth fine lines, but mostly they will help to polish and brighten your skin.

Prevent

Morning. Ideally, your moisturizer contains sunscreen. However, if it doesn't, or if you're going to be outside for much of the day, apply a good-quality, broad-spectrum sunscreen (one that shields you from both UVA and UVB rays) to *all* areas of the skin that will be exposed to the sun. Then reapply it every few hours that you remain outside. (See pages 103–106 for more information on sunscreens.) Keep in mind that it takes about one ounce (or a full shot glass) of the stuff to cover your entire body. Studies show that an SPF 30 sunscreen, applied in the quantities that most people use, yields an SPF of only about 2. During the week, or on days when your outdoor activities are limited, you should use a combination product that contains a sunscreen and anti-aging ingredients. Reapplication on these days is less important.

Dr. Dover Recommends

Drugstore

- Skin Effects Sun Effects Active SPF 45
- Olay Complete Touch of Sun Daily UV Facial Moisturizer
- Neutrogena Ultra Sheer Dry-Touch Sunblock with Helioplex, SPF 55

Department Store and Doctor's Office

- N.V. Perricone M.D. Solar Protection for Face SPF 26
- Sisley Broad Spectrum Sunscreen SPF 40, Colorless

Ellen's Story: Looking Old Overnight

Ellen was in the women's bathroom of an exclusive restaurant when she first noticed how old her eyes had become—seemingly overnight. The forty-four-year-old Pilates instructor had always taken pride in the fact that she looked far younger than her age, or so her friends told her. Suddenly, it seemed, the crow's feet extending from her eyes were especially obvious. They made her entire face look tired and old.

Ellen had several friends who regularly booked Botox appointments, so she knew how safe and surprisingly affordable these treatments are. However, she was the natural type, and she wanted to rely on topicals for as long as possible. I was frank with Ellen. I told her that not even the best cream—including the ones that billed themselves as needle-free alternatives to Botox—would obliterate the lines around her eyes, which were etched into her skin like pleats in a pair of pants. Nevertheless, there were ways to make the area look tighter and smoother.

I suggested that she toss out the drying cleanser that she had been using on her face since her twenties; it was just zapping moisture from her skin, making any lines look more obvious. By simply switching to a creamier wash with fewer surfactants (or detergents) and adding a rich nighttime moisturizer, Ellen would draw water into her skin, plumping it up and making it look smoother instantly. For long-term change, I advised her to choose an eye cream with line-smoothing retinol and peptides to help build collagen, along with a skin-tightening ingredient like DMAE, GABA, or lycopene. To keep her eyes and the rest of her face looking as smooth as possible, I prescribed a retinoid and told her to begin using it only every other night until her skin grew accustomed to it.

This skin-care regimen would improve Ellen's overall skin quality, moisture content, texture, and tone and would smooth out fine wrinkles, but it would do little for the actual creases around her eyes. For these I suggested that she consider Botox in the future.

Six weeks later, the skin-care regimen had made a difference in the fine crinkles around her eyes; they had softened a bit, and her face as a whole looked much softer, brighter, fresher, and younger. She knows that she can always turn to Botox later to keep the creases permanently at bay, but the topical plan she's following now will continue to improve her overall skin for months—and years—to come.

A Skin-Care Regimen for Your SVA: Fifties

What you see in the mirror: a complexion that looks drier, duller, and more tired because of age, sun, and hormonal shifts. At the same time, redness and the blood vessels in the cheeks and around the nose might be more apparent. Sun-induced brown spots increase in number and size. Forehead lines and crow's feet deepen, and volume loss extends to the rest of the face, the neck, and other parts of the body, leading to more sagging and sometimes, around the eyes, hollowness. Other areas, like the neck, the belly, the hips, and the buttocks, tend to accumulate fat with age.

Cleanse

Morning and night. Wash with your favorite cleanser. Switching to a creamier formula will help your skin to hold on to its own fatty acids, which give your face a natural glow and plumpness. (See page 41 for specific types of cleansers.)

Dr. Dover Recommends

Drugstore

- Skin Effects Gentle Foaming Cleanser
- Eucerin Gentle Hydrating Cleanser
- Neutrogena Extra Gentle Cleanser, Fragrance Free

Department Store and Doctor's Office
- RéVive Cleanser Crème Luxe
- Dr. Brandt Lineless Gel Cleanser

To further boost your skin's radiance and to speed up your increasingly sluggish cell turnover, treat your complexion to an exfoliating scrub two or three times a week. Choose either a physical formula that contains round, soft grains or a chemical one with alpha hydroxy acid or fruit enzymes. Exfoliating increases the penetration of whatever cream or lotion you apply immediately after, so it's best to exfoliate at night before moving on to the "treat" step.

Dr. Dover Recommends

Drugstore

- Skin Effects Deep Cleaning Enzyme Scrub or Self-Heating Resurfacing Cleanser
- RoC Age Diminishing Facial Cleanser

- Neutrogena Healthy Skin Visibly Even Skin Polishing Enzyme Treatment
- Olay Regenerist Microdermabrasion and Peel System

Department Store and Doctor's Office
- Patricia Wexler M.D. Dermatology Dual Action Foaming Cleanser
- Clé de Peau Refreshing Cleansing Foam

Treat

Morning. Start with a skin-brightening product that contains an ingredient like hydroquinone, kojic acid, soy, Sepiwhite MSH, or green or black tea to combat your sun-induced brown spots and to help brighten your skin.

Dr. Dover Recommends

Drugstore
- Skin Effects Advanced Brightening Complex
- La Roche-Posay Mela-D Skin Lightening Daily Lotion
- Aveeno Active Naturals Positively Radiant Eye Brightening Cream

Department Store and Doctor's Office
- DDF Intensive Holistic Lightener
- Dr. Brandt Laser Lightening Day Lotion

Apply a moisturizer that will also work on wrinkles and dulling skin; it's even better if it contains sunscreen. Some of my favorites have hydrating ingredients, like hyaluronic acid and glycerin; anti-aging ingredients, like glycolic acid, peptides, and vitamins A (retinol, retinyl palmitate), C (ascorbic acid, ascorbyl palmitate), and E (tocopheryl); and antioxidants, like vitamin C, green tea, coenzyme Q10, or idebenone. The antioxidants will help to mop up damaging free radicals that the skin has generated in response to sun exposure, pollutants, and other environmental factors.

Dr. Dover Recommends

Drugstore

- Skin Effects Redness Control Daily Moisturizer SPF 30+
- Neutrogena Anti-Oxidant Age Reverse Day Lotion SPF 20

Department Store and Doctor's Office

- Kinerase Ultimate Day Moisturizer
- La Mer The Concentrate

Night. If you haven't already done so, ask your dermatologist to prescribe a retinoid cream to speed sluggish cell turnover, increase collagen production, and help the skin to look and feel younger. Depending on which retinoid you use, you might notice that your complexion feels drier, especially during the first few weeks of use. Applying a night moisturizer five minutes after putting on your retinoid will help. (See pages 59–63 for information on retinoids.)

After putting on the prescription retinoid, lightly coat both the face and the neck with a skin-firming product. Look for formulas with tightening ingredients like GABA, lycopene, DMAE, or alpha lipoic acid.

Dr. Dover Recommends

Drugstore

- Skin Effects Firming Face and Neck Cream
- Olay Total Effects Night Firming Cream for Face & Neck
- Vichy LiftActiv Pro Night Detoxifying Anti-Wrinkle and Firming Care

Department Store and Doctor's Office

- N.V. Perricone M.D. Neuropeptide Facial Conformer
- DDF Bio-Molecular Firming Eye Serum

Apply an eye cream that contains rich moisturizers, like glycerin, cyclopentasiloxane, silicone, and dimethicone, as well as brighteners, like vitamin C derivatives and licorice extract (glycerrhetinic acid). If fine lines surrounding the eyes are a problem, be sure that your cream has vitamin A. If you're suffering from puffiness around the eyes, look for a cream with caffeine and alpha lipoic acid.

Dr. Dover Recommends

Drugstore

- Skin Effects Dual Action Under Eye Therapy
- RoC Retin-OL Multi-Correxion Eye
- La Roche-Posay Hydraphase Eyes
- Olay Regenerist Eye Derma-Pod Anti-Aging Triple Response System

Department Store and Doctor's Office

- N.V. Perricone M.D. Advanced Eye Area Therapy
- Patricia Wexler M.D. Instant De-Puff Eye Gel
- Orlane Hypnotherapy Eye Cream

Extra credit: night. If your skin is starting to feel more parched than usual, adding a heavier night cream—a moisturizer that's slightly richer than daytime formulas and, of course, doesn't have sunscreen—will make your complexion look more plump and dewy when you wake up. There's no reason not to choose a formula containing anti-aging components.

Dr. Dover Recommends

Drugstore

- Skin Effects Cell 2 Cell Continuous Action Anti-Wrinkle Care followed by a layer of Skin Effects Intensive Overnight Repair Cream
- Olay Age Defying Anti-Wrinkle Replenishing Night Cream
- Eucerin Plus Intensive Repair Lotion with Alpha Hydroxyl

Department Store and Doctor's Office

- DDF Cellular Revitalization Age Renewal
- Kinerase Pro+ Therapy Cream with Kinetin & Zeatin
- Clé de Peau Enriched Nourishing Cream

Add a topical growth factor, a class of anti-aging ingredients derived from many of the compounds that are found in healthy newborn skin and are responsible for healing wounds and producing new skin cells.

Dr. Dover Recommends

Department Store and Doctor's Office
- SkinMedica TNS Dermal Repair Cream
- Neocutis Hyalis 1% Hyaluronate Refining Serum

Anytime. Occasionally, book a series of light glycolic acid peels, microdermabrasion, or a vibraderm treatment. Performed in a dermatologist's office or in a doctor-supervised medical spa, these procedures encourage deeper cell turnover, cause brown spots to fade, and smooth fine lines, but mostly they will help to polish and brighten your skin.

Prevent

Morning. Ideally, your moisturizer contains sunscreen. However, if it doesn't, or if you're going to be outside for much of the day, apply a good-quality, broad-spectrum sunscreen (one that shields you from both UVA and UVB rays) to *all* areas of the skin that will be exposed to the sun. Then reapply it every few hours that you remain outside. (See pages 103–106 for more information on sunscreens.) Keep in mind that it takes about one ounce (or a full shot glass) of the stuff to cover your entire body. Studies show that an SPF 30 sunscreen, applied in the quantities that most people use, yields an SPF of only about 2. During the week, or on days when your outdoor activities are limited, you should use a combination product that contains a sunscreen and anti-aging ingredients. Reapplication on these days is less important.

Dr. Dover Recommends

Drugstore
- Skin Effects Sun Effects Continuous Spray SPF Active Sunscreen 45

- La Roche-Posay Biomedic Facial Shield SPF 20
- Neutrogena Ultra Sheer Dry-Touch Sunblock with Helioplex, SPF 55

Department Store and Doctor's Office
- Dr. Brandt Daily UV Protection SPF 30 Colorless
- Orlane Anti-Wrinkle Sun Serum for the Face

Ruth's Story: The Power of Creams

"Dr. Dover, I just don't *feel* this old," said Ruth when she came in to see me last year. At age fifty-eight, she was clearly in the prime of her life: working as a gallery curator and spending weekends going on long bike rides with her husband and chasing her young grandchildren around the house. Recently, however, whenever Ruth looked in the mirror, she was seeing someone who was beginning to resemble the grandmother she remembered as a child, and she wasn't happy about it.

Although her face was still mostly free of wrinkles, Ruth was troubled by the crepelike texture of her skin, the fine lines, the uneven pigmentation, and the facial sagging. For years, she had been doing a very simple skin-care regimen. She washed her face morning and night, then used a beautifully packaged, $200-a-jar moisturizer and night cream that she bought at a high-end department store. Although it smelled fantastic and had great texture, it was doing little to make her actually look younger. The first thing I did was to steer her away from her overpriced creams and suggest a more effective—not to mention less expensive—cream that contains moisturizers, anti-aging ingredients, and sunscreen for her to use in the morning. I also recommended a similar but richer cream without sunscreen for night use. Then I went to work on a long-term plan that would coax her skin's collagen production to go into overdrive: a prescription retinoid cream paired with a serum that contains growth factors. These two products are not inexpensive, but both were still less costly than her department store cream and much more effective as well.

Ruth was dubious at first, but she decided to try my plan for a month, and she was delighted when she began to notice a difference. She continued with it for another month and was overjoyed at how much creamier her complexion had suddenly become. For the first time in a few years, Ruth looks almost as young as she feels.

A Skin-Care Regimen for Your SVA: Sixties

What you see in the mirror: a complexion that reflects decades of bad habits—and we all have them. Perhaps you spent your young adulthood sunning yourself every weekend, subjected your rosacea-prone skin to too much red wine, or smoked cigarettes against your better judgment. Or perhaps you've simply neglected your skin. Regardless, your cheeks are likely to be more ruddy, your lines are too dramatic to smooth away with an ordinary moisturizer, and your skin continues to sag. Meanwhile, the fat padding your belly, hips, and buttocks isn't going anywhere.

Cleanse

Morning and night. Wash with your favorite cleanser. Switching to a creamier formula will help your skin to hold onto its own fatty acids, which give your face a natural glow and plumpness. (See page 41 for specific types of cleansers.)

Dr. Dover Recommends

Drugstore

- Skin Effects Gentle Foaming Cleanser
- Olay Foaming Face Wash for Sensitive Skin
- Cetaphil Gentle Skin Cleanser
- La Roche-Posay Lipikar Surgras Cleansing Bar

Department Store and Doctor's Office

- SkinMedica Sensitive Skin Cleanser
- N.V. Perricone M.D. Vitamin C Ester Citrus Facial Wash

To further boost your skin's radiance and to speed up your increasingly sluggish cell turnover, treat your complexion to an exfoliating scrub two or three times a week. Choose either a physical formula that contains round soft grains or a chemical one with alpha hydroxy acid or fruit enzymes. Exfoliating increases the penetration of whatever cream or lotion you apply immediately after, so it's best to exfoliate at night before moving on to the "treat" step.

Dr. Dover Recommends

Drugstore

- Skin Effects Deep Cleaning Enzyme Scrub
- RoC Age Diminishing Facial Cleanser
- La Roche-Posay Biomedic Micro Exfoliating Scrub

Department Store and Doctor's Office

- DDF Glycolic 5% Daily Cleansing Pads
- Clé de Peau Refreshing Cleansing Foam

Treat

Morning. Start with a skin-brightening product that contains an ingredient like hydroquinone, kojic acid, soy, Sepiwhite MSH, or green or black tea to combat your sun-induced brown spots and to help brighten your skin.

Dr. Dover Recommends

Drugstore

- Skin Effects Advanced Brightening Complex
- Neutrogena Illuminating Whip Moisturizer

Department Store and Doctor's Office

- N.V. Perricone M.D. Advanced Face Firming Activator
- La Prairie Cellular Anti-Spot Brightening Serum

Apply a moisturizer that will also work on wrinkles and dulling skin; it's even better if it contains sunscreen. Some of my favorites contain hydrating ingredients, like hyaluronic acid and glycerin; anti-aging ingredients, like glycolic acid, peptides, and vitamins A (retinol, retinyl palmitate), C (ascorbic acid, ascorbyl palmitate), and E (tocopheryl); and antioxidants, like vitamin C, green tea, coenzyme Q10, or idebenone.

Dr. Dover Recommends

Drugstore
- Skin Effects Cell 2 Cell Continuous Action Anti-Wrinkle Care
- Skin Effects Preventing Effects Lightweight Moisturizing Soufflé
- RoC Age Diminishing Daily Moisturizer SPF 15
- Aveeno Positively Ageless Daily Moisturizer SPF 30 UVA/UVB

Department Store and Doctor's Office
- Cellex-C Skin Firming Cream Plus
- La Prairie Anti-Aging Stress Cream

Night. By now, I hope you're using a retinoid cream regularly to speed sluggish cell turnover, increase collagen production, and help the skin to look and feel younger. (See pages 59–63 for information on retinoids.) If you haven't yet switched to a creamier formula, like Renova, to help the skin retain its moisture, this is a great time to do so.

After putting on the retinoid cream, lightly coat both the face and the neck with a skin-firming product. Look for formulas with tightening ingredients like lycopene or DMAE.

Dr. Dover Recommends

Drugstore
- Skin Effects 7 Day Firming Program
- RoC Protient Lift and Define Serum

Department Store and Doctor's Office
- Clé de Peau Facial Contour Treatment Set
- Crème de la Mer

Apply an eye cream that contains rich moisturizers, like glycerin, cyclopentasiloxane, silicone, and dimethicone, as well as brighteners, like vitamin C derivatives and licorice extract (glycerrhetinic acid). If fine lines surrounding the eyes are a problem, be sure that your cream has vitamin A. If you're suffering from puffiness around the eyes, look for a cream with caffeine and alpha lipoic acid.

Dr. Dover Recommends

Drugstore
- Skin Effects Dual Action Under Eye Therapy
- Olay Total Effects Eye Transforming Cream with VitaNiacin
- Neutrogena Radiance Boost Eye Cream

Department Store and Doctor's Office
- SkinCare Prescription Anti-Aging Eye Cream
- SkinMedica TNS Illuminating Eye Cream
- La Mer The Eye Balm

If your skin is starting to feel more parched than usual, adding a heavier night cream—a moisturizer that's slightly richer than daytime formulas and, of course, doesn't have sunscreen—will make your complexion look more plump and dewy when you wake up. There's no reason not to choose a formula that contains anti-aging components.

Dr. Dover Recommends

Drugstore
- Skin Effects Intensive Overnight Repair Cream
- Neutrogena Anti-Oxidant Age Reverse Night Cream
- La Roche-Posay Active C Anti-Wrinkle Dermatological Treatment Day/Night Emulsion

Department Store and Doctor's Office
- SkinCare Prescription Night Anti-Aging Moisturizer with Retinol
- Prevage Anti-Aging Night Cream

Add a topical growth factor, a class of anti-aging ingredients derived from many of the compounds that are found in healthy newborn skin and are responsible for healing wounds and producing new skin cells.

Dr. Dover Recommends

Department Store and Doctor's Office
- SkinMedica TNS Hydrating Masque
- RéVive Intensité Crème Lustre

Anytime. Occasionally, book a series of glycolic acid peels, microdermabrasion, or a vibraderm treatment. Performed in a dermatologist's office or in a doctor-supervised medical spa, these procedures encourage deeper cell turnover, cause brown spots to fade, and smooth fine lines, but mostly they will help to polish and brighten your skin.

Prevent

Morning. Ideally, your moisturizer contains sunscreen. However, if it doesn't, or if you're going to be outside for much of the day, apply a good-quality, broad-spectrum sunscreen (one that shields you from both UVA and UVB rays) to *all* areas of the skin that will be exposed to the sun. Then reapply it every few hours that you remain outside. (See pages 103–106 for more information on sunscreens.) Keep in mind that it takes about one ounce (or a full shot glass) of the stuff to cover your entire body. Studies show that an SPF 30 sunscreen, applied in the quantities that most people use, yields an SPF of only about 2. During the week, or on days when your outdoor activities are limited, you should use a combination product that contains a sunscreen and anti-aging ingredients. Reapplication on these days is less important.

Dr. Dover Recommends

Drugstore

- Skin Effects Sun Effects Active SPF 45
- Neutrogena Sensitive Skin Sunblock Lotion SPF 30
- Neutrogena Ultra Soft Hydrating Sunblock, SPF 45
- Vichy Capital Soleil SPF 15 Sunscreen Cream with Mexoryl SX

Department Store and Doctor's Office

- DDF Organic Sunblock SPF 30
- Dr. Brandt Daily UV Protection SPF 30 Face, in light bronze or medium bronze

Evelyn's Story: Refreshing Her Skin after Menopause

Any dermatologist would say that Evelyn did everything right. She had been washing her face with a cleanser and wearing sunscreen dutifully since her early twenties. When alpha hydroxy acids came on the scene in the early 1990s, she began using a glycolic lotion to lift away dead skin cells. Since her mid-forties, she had been using a powerful prescription retinoid I had prescribed for her.

This is why, at age sixty, Evelyn had the skin of someone a decade younger. During the last several years, however, her skin had begun to look more haggard and dry—a change she rightfully associated with the onset of menopause. For many women, a drop in estrogen causes a number of changes in the skin, including a decreased production of oil, which means that products you relied on for years suddenly feel harsh and often leave your complexion parched, flaky, and sometimes irritated. In response, Evelyn had stopped applying her retinoid cream and was using only a basic moisturizer morning and night.

I certainly understood her inclination. Who wants to have fewer lines if it also means having red, scaly patches? In fact, retinoid-induced dry skin looks *more* wrinkled, not less. However, I urged

Evelyn not to give up on retinoids yet. These powerful vitamin A derivatives are truly the gold standard in anti-aging topicals. Instead, I said, she simply had to find the *right* retinoid to suit her changing skin, and then use it properly. I sent her home with a sample tube of one of the creamier formulas, Renova, to help rejuvenate her skin while also replenishing some of its lost moisture. I asked her to apply a rich night cream on top, which made her complexion look dewier and younger overnight, then I tracked down a luscious, soufflé-like cleanser to replace her harsher foaming version. Less than two months later, Evelyn's skin had noticeably more bounce and luster, with not a dry patch or a flake in sight.

A Skin-Care Regimen for Your SVA: Seventies and Beyond

What you see in the mirror: increasing dullness, redness, and brown spots, along with a pattern of creases and folds between the brows, running from the nose to the mouth, lining the upper lip, and extending down from the crow's feet to along the cheeks. Meanwhile, the skin continues to droop, especially around the forehead, the jawline, and the neck, but also over the rest of the body. Since no topical product will be able to remedy these issues overnight, or even over several weeks or months, this is when your skin-care history really starts to catch up with you. The key now is to include as many active ingredients as possible in every part of your regimen.

Cleanse

Morning and night. Switching to a creamier cleanser will help your skin to hold on to its own fatty acids and to keep in as much of its natural moisture as possible. (See page 41 for specific types of cleansers.)

Dr. Dover Recommends

Drugstore
- Vichy Detoxifying Cleansing Milk

- La Roche-Posay Toleriane Gentle Cleansing Bar
- Dove Beauty Bar

Department Store and Doctor's Office

- Patricia Wexler M.D. Dermatology Universal Anti-Aging Cleanser
- Sisley Botanical Soapless Facial Cleansing Bar

Treat

Morning. Be sure to use creams rather than lotions. In general, you should be choosing the most moisturizing products available. Use a creamy moisturizer that contains both anti-aging ingredients and a sunscreen.

Dr. Dover Recommends

Drugstore

- Skin Effects Cell 2 Cell Continuous Action Anti-Wrinkle Care
- Skin Effects Preventing Effects Lightweight Moisturizing Soufflé
- Skin Effects Daily Anti-Aging Treatment Cream SPF 15
- RoC Deep Wrinkle Daily Moisturizer SPF 15
- Eucerin Q10 Anti-Wrinkle Sensitive Skin Crème and Lotion SPF 15

Department Store and Doctor's Office

- Patricia Wexler M.D. Dermatology Universal Anti-Aging Moisturizer SPF 30+
- RéVive Moisturizing Renewal Cream

Night. Absolutely use a prescription retinoid—but make sure it's a creamier version, like Renova, which helps the skin to retain its moisture while it rejuvenates the skin.

After putting on the prescription retinoid cream, lightly coat both the face and the neck with a skin-firming product. Look for formulas with tightening ingredients like GABA, lycopene, DMAE, or alpha lipoic acid.

Dr. Dover Recommends

Drugstore
- Skin Effects Intense 7 Day Firming Program
- La Roche-Posay Redermic Daily Fill-in Anti-Wrinkle Firming Care for Dry Skin
- Vichy NeOvadiol Intensive Crease Smoothing Densifying Care

Department Store and Doctor's Office
- Dr. Brandt r3p Cream
- SkinCeuticals Renew Overnight Dry Nighttime Skin-Refining Moisturizer for Normal or Dry Skin

Apply an eye cream that contains rich moisturizers, like glycerin, as well as brighteners, like vitamin C derivatives and licorice extract (glycerrhetinic acid). If fine lines surrounding the eyes are a problem, be sure that your cream has vitamin A. If you're suffering from puffiness around the eyes, look for a formula with caffeine and alpha lipoic acid.

Dr. Dover Recommends

Drugstore
- Skin Effects Dual Action Under Eye Therapy
- RoC Protient Fortify Lift and Define Eye Cream
- La Roche-Posay Redermic Eyes

Department Store and Doctor's Office
- SkinCare Prescription Anti-Aging Eye Cream
- N.V. Perricone M.D. Neuropeptide Eye Area Contour
- Patricia Wexler M.D. Dermatology Fastscription No-Injection Instant Line Filler for Lips & Eyes
- La Prairie Cellular Radiance Eye Cream

If your skin is starting to feel more parched than usual, adding a heavier night cream—a moisturizer that's slightly richer than daytime formulas and, of course, doesn't have sunscreen—will make your complexion look more plump and dewy when you wake up. There's no reason not to choose a formula that contains anti-aging components.

Dr. Dover Recommends

Drugstore

- Skin Effects Intensive Overnight Repair Cream
- Skin Effects Skin Quenching Daily Mask
- Olay Complete Night Fortifying Cream
- RoC Retinol Correxion Deep Wrinkle Night Cream
- Olay Regenerist Deep Hydration Regenerating Cream

Department Store and Doctor's Office

- Patricia Wexler M.D. Dermatology Intensive Night Reversal & Repair Cream
- Orlane Absolute Skin Recovery Repairing Night Cream

Add a topical growth factor, a class of anti-aging ingredients derived from many of the compounds that are found in healthy newborn skin and are responsible for healing wounds and producing new skin cells.

Dr. Dover Recommends

Department Store and Doctor's Office

- SkinMedica TNS Ceramide Treatment Cream
- Neocutis Bio-Gel Bio-Restorative Hydrogel

Anytime. Occasionally, see a medical aesthetician, preferably at your dermatologist's office or at a medical spa under the supervision of a dermatologist or a plastic surgeon. He or she can tailor a program for older, sun-damaged, sensitive skin that will help to bring the glow and a softer feel back to your complexion. This might include a medical cleansing and a series of gentle peels.

Prevent

Morning. Ideally, your moisturizer contains sunscreen. However, if it doesn't, or if you're going to be outside for much of the day, apply a good-quality, broad-spectrum sunscreen (one that shields you from both UVA and UVB rays) to *all* areas of the skin that will be exposed to the sun. Then reapply it every few hours that you remain outside. (See pages 103–106 for more information on sunscreens.) Keep in mind that it takes about one ounce (or a full shot glass) of the stuff to cover your entire body. Studies show that an SPF 30 sunscreen, applied in the quantities that most people use, yields an SPF of only about 2. During the week, or on days when your outdoor activities are limited, you should use a combination product that contains a sunscreen and anti-aging ingredients. Reapplication on these days is less important.

Dr. Dover Recommends

Drugstore
- Skin Effects Preventing Effects Lightweight Moisturizing Soufflé SPF 30
- Skin Effects Sun Effects Active SPF 45
- Olay Definity Correcting Protective Lotion with SPF 15
- La Roche-Posay Anthelios 40 Sunscreen Cream with Mexoryl SX

Department Store and Doctor's Office
- La Mer The SPF 18 Fluid
- Sisley Broad-Spectrum Sunscreen SPF 25-Amber

Rose's Story: Reducing Her SVA at Age Seventy-Six

The first thing that Rose pointed out to me during our first chat was her skin's dry, saggy appearance. The seventy-six-year-old retired travel agent was troubled by her skin's loss of elasticity, and she hated the fact that she looked perpetually tired. Then she hesitantly told me what upset her most of all: "My granddaughter won't sit on my lap because she's afraid of the way I look," she said.

Rose assumed that there was nothing she could do, short of surgery—which was definitely *not* in her plans—to turn her skin around. I couldn't lie to her: no cream or skin-care regimen would work miracles at this point, after years of sun damage had accumulated on her face. Nevertheless, the right products could definitely make a significant difference. I started by giving Rose a sample of a thick, lipid-rich cleanser. Since she had been using a drying, foamy wash, replenishing her skin's own fatty acids immediately made her face look more vibrant and hydrated, which minimized the appearance of her fine lines. I told her to swap all her treatment lotions for cream versions and to look for a morning moisturizer that also contained anti-aging ingredients like glycolic acid and vitamin C.

Rose had never used a retinoid before, and I knew that just six weeks of applying one would make her skin look younger, so I prescribed one of the creamiest formulas, Renova, for bedtime and suggested that she layer a skin-firming cream over it along with a growth factor cream and a brightening eye cream. A month and a half of this treatment didn't work miracles, but it did work wonders. Her face looks more refreshed, tighter, and radiant. "I'm ecstatic," Rose told me on our follow-up visit, as her granddaughter snuggled happily into her lap.

Doctor's Orders

Once I've sent my patients home with a skin-care regimen, many of them end up sitting in front of their vanity mirror, staring at their new products, and wondering exactly how to apply them. How long after cleansing the face should the first treatment cream be applied? When there are multiple products in the regimen, which ones should be used when, and how exactly should they be layered? These are excellent questions. The application technique that you use for these potions and lotions really can make a difference in how well or how poorly they work. Here are some of my favorite tips:

Start clean. It might sound elementary to say that you should wash your face first, but you'd be surprised how many people slather on treatment products without doing that. The more gunk your lotion or cream has to penetrate before going to work on your trouble spots, the less effective it will be. So begin with a clean canvas: a face free of makeup, oil, and dirt.

Slough away the rough spots. This step is optional, but using an exfoliating cleanser—a physical formula that contains gentle scrubbing beads or a chemical formula with a very mild acid or enzymes—will break down the uppermost layer of dead skin cells, further enabling your treatment product to penetrate deeply.

Dry off. Pat your face dry, then move on immediately to the next step—unless you're using a prescription retinoid. Since that can be irritating if used on damp skin, be sure to wait at least five minutes (up to thirty minutes if you have very sensitive skin) after washing before you apply a retinoid.

Establish order. Many of my patients, especially those with more mature skin, are juggling several treatment products. The best rule for layering them is as follows: start with the thinnest formula and end with the thickest. Gels always go on before serums, serums before lotions, and lotions before creams. (I hope, however, that you won't be using *quite* so many products!)

Don't sweat the small stuff. Despite what you might have heard, using a fancy application technique, like semicircular motions, won't help your treatment product to work any better. Just rub it on gently, covering the entire face (or the areas you'd like to treat) with a very light film. *Over*applying won't make the formula work any faster. Finally, be careful not to use too many irritating items. Prescription retinoids, brightening creams with 4 percent or higher hydroquinone, and some acne products can be harsh, especially when they are layered on top of one another.

part three

beyond topicals

Clearly, choosing the right creams, lotions, and serums for your skin and its virtual age can do wonders for your complexion. As a dermatologist, I'm thrilled to see the myriad of truly effective at-home and in-office treatments that are available now. Many of them have the power to slow the aging process, smooth away existing fine lines, and cause brown spots to fade over time.

The operative words here are *over time.* A topical cream or a minor in-office peel almost always costs less than the more aggressive procedures that we dermatologists have at our disposal. Sometimes, however, you just don't want to wait weeks, months, or even years to see a significant change in your SVA. Perhaps you have a major event coming up; perhaps you've simply stared at your crow's feet or frown lines or age spots long enough. Either way, there's good news for those who want to be more proactive about knocking years off their faces.

My office is filled with treatments that will obliterate lines and creases, zap unwanted spots, and tighten sagging skin remarkably well. We have injectable fillers, wrinkle-relaxing substances, lasers, and energy-source devices that take less time than a long business lunch and require only a minimal recovery period, so you can usually return to your normal life that afternoon or the very next day. Best of all, as high-tech and fast-acting as these treatments are, they're not nearly as costly as you might think, especially when you consider that you might be able to eliminate some of the fancier, costlier creams from your daily regimen.

For those who want to accelerate the battle against aging one more level, cosmetic surgery is always an option. A good dermatologist not only helps a patient to reach his or her goal, he or she also determines whether that patient should consider surgery. Thus, I'll spend the last chapter of this section outlining some of the most popular surgical procedures and offering ways to determine which ones, if any, are right for you.

Regardless of how much a doctor can tighten, smooth, or lift your skin, you must still keep it clean, encourage healthy cell turnover, reverse existing sun damage, and prevent new damage on a daily basis. Thus, even if you ultimately decide to take a more aggressive approach toward anti-aging—whether by booking a Botox or a filler visit, scheduling a laser consultation, or investigating eye-lift surgery—good topical skin care should still always play a key role. This will help to preserve the results of those in-office treatments and will keep your SVA from creeping back up.

7

Injection Options

W hen I mention the words *filler* or *Botox* to my patients, some bristle at first. Many of them are exceedingly down-to-earth people who would never dream of using anything stronger than a prescription retinoid to smooth their fine lines and cause their brown spots to fade. When certain areas of the face begin to sag, crease, or wrinkle, at least some of them are determined to accept the change gracefully. They're happy to use face cream, but the thought of anything more than that scares them or doesn't suit their personalities. Of course, there's nothing wrong with feeling this way, especially because we have so many highly effective topical products at our disposal these days.

Neverthless, the increasing availability of injectables, like Botox and fillers—and the fact that dermatologists are more adept than ever at using them—has made it easy, safe, and cost-effective for people to make immediate, natural-looking changes without spending an exorbitant amount of money. Let's start by determining how much *you* know about the vast and growing world of injectables.

1. Which of the following is a true statement about Botox?
    A. It's safe when used by a physician or a trained practitioner who is supervised by a physician.
    B. It's safe anytime—including when used in spas, salons, and "Botox parties."
    C. It is dangerous and is best avoided.

2. The effects of a single Botox treatment last for approximately
    A. One month
    B. Three to four months
    C. Forever

3. What is the best age to start using Botox?
    A. My forties or earlier
    B. My fifties or later
    C. There is no set age

5. The most popular injectable fillers contain
    A. Collagen
    B. Hyaluronic acid fillers, like Restylane and Juvederm
    C. Silicone

5. Which of the following is Botox not able to do?
    A. Smooth forehead lines
    B. Minimize excessive sweating on the palms and other areas of the body
    C. Lift my eyebrows slightly
    D. Get rid of cellulite

6. The most effective treatment for crow's feet is
    A. Botox
    B. Fillers, like collagen and hyaluronic acid
    C. A really good wrinkle cream, like Retin-A

7. When choosing a filler, which kind should I select?
    A. One that lasts as long as possible—a permanent filler is ideal
    B. One that lasts several months
    C. It depends on my lifestyle and on the areas I'd like to address.

8. Fillers and Botox used for "off-label" purposes
   A. Are illegal—stay away from them at all costs
   B. Have been FDA-approved for some uses but not for others
   C. Are perfectly safe for any use

9. People who use Botox and fillers together to both relax *and* fill a crease or a fold
   A. Usually see even better results than if they were to use only one of those treatments
   B. Are spending twice as much on a treatment than they need to spend
   C. Are taking an unnecessary risk

10. A bit of swelling after a filler injection is
    A. Normal; certain fillers lead to more swelling than others
    B. A sign of poor technique; find a new dermatologist
    C. Always a red flag; seek medical help immediately

Answers

1. A: Doctors have been using Botox for decades, and it's been approved for the cosmetic treatment of frown lines for more than ten years. The drug is extremely safe—when used in expert hands. Since injecting Botox is an art as well as a science, it's best to go to an experienced dermatologist or plastic surgeon or to a practitioner supervised by one.

2. B: The effect of a Botox treatment peaks about ten days after the injection and gradually fades three to four months later.

3. C: Rather than focusing on your chronological age, let your SVA guide you. If you're bothered by lines or wrinkles on your face, it makes perfect sense to talk to your doctor about Botox. There's even evidence to show that starting Botox before dramatic creases and frown lines appear can prevent them from ever forming.

4. B: Collagen was the original and only filler available in the United States for decades, but hyaluronic acid has recently

surpassed collagen in popularity. Since hyaluronic acid comes in many different consistencies, it's a great option for filling many different areas on the face. Silicone is a much more controversial filler, mostly because it lasts forever.

5. D: Botox is truly a wonderful treatment for all kinds of issues. It can minimize excess sweating and even lift the brows ever so slightly. Alas, Botox cannot do anything for cellulite, which is notoriously resistant to a variety of treatments.

6. A: Although fillers do a great job of smoothing out fine lines and deeper wrinkles, they're best used for folds rather than creases. Botox is the treatment of choice for what dermatologists call the "lines of negative facial expression" or for the lines caused by muscular activity, such as crow's feet. A good-quality wrinkle cream can absolutely help to minimize fine lines and very early crow's feet, but the improvements will be far more gradual and less dramatic than with Botox.

7. C: Many people erroneously assume that permanent fillers are always a better bet, but what if you're not happy with your results? Suppose you decide sometime later that you'd like your lips to be a bit less pillowy than they've been for the past several years? Permanent fillers also have permanent side effects. Choosing a filler is a very personal decision, which a good doctor can help you to make.

8. B: An off-label treatment is one that uses an existing FDA-approved product for a use that is different from the one for which the product was originally approved. For instance, Botox is approved for cosmetic treatment of frown lines between the brows but not for crow's feet or forehead creases and lines. Off-label treatments are not necessarily dangerous. The company that makes the product has simply not submitted the safety and effectiveness data for that alternative purpose to the FDA. If you're going to use Botox for an off-label treatment, it's crucial to see an experienced doctor you trust.

9. A: A Botox-filler combination therapy is actually one of the most effective, underrated ways to treat the deep creases between the brows. The two injectables work synergistically, each prolonging the life span of the other, with spectacular results.

10. A: Certain fillers, like Restylane, often cause minor swelling that can be a bit unsightly for a day or so but is otherwise perfectly normal. Allergic reactions to most fillers are now rare, but if you believe you're having such a reaction, contact your doctor immediately.

Cleansers, lotions, and creams are the staples of my patients' treatment regimens. In spite of all the high-tech advanced ingredients that are designed to make the skin look and feel as if it were years younger, I still spend time during every patient visit reviewing the simple skin-care regimens that require only a few dabs and a few minutes every morning and evening in front of the bathroom mirror. The right topical skin-care routine can make a world of difference to your SVA.

Sometimes, however, you want to go beyond the basic staples. When the wrinkles and crinkles are too deep for even the best topicals to handle—or when you don't want to wait the weeks or months they can take to work—you might choose to add a more aggressive treatment into the mix. Remember Jessica? She was the thirty-six-year-old mother of two who walked into my office a few months before her college reunion after catching sight of her deepening lines in one of those unflattering dressing-room mirrors. I wound up sending her home with a skin-care regimen that included a prescription for Retin-A, which has done wonders for her skin's texture and tone.

Here's what I didn't mention earlier: during that first consultation with Jessica, I started by giving her a large hand mirror and asking her to explain what bothered her; after all, she knows her own skin better than I do. Like many women, Jessica could live with the crinkles around her eyes, because at least they're usually accompanied by a smile. The only thing she mentioned that bothered her was the lack of overall luster that she thought made her face look tired.

We spent most of the fifteen-minute visit talking about skin care: the prescription retinoids, sunscreen, glycolic peels, and microderm-abrasion that would slowly restore some of that lost luster and begin to smooth away her finest lines. Then, as were finishing, she said, "You know, doctor, this has been really helpful, but I'm surprised you didn't mention Botox." I can't tell you how often I hear this from patients. Botox has become so popular that it's the rare patient of mine who has not heard of it and wondered if it is right for him or her. Many individuals are looking to give their topical routine a little kick-start; or, like Jessica, they wish for a treatment that will work quickly enough for a college reunion.

It turns out that Jessica was bothered by the shallow frown lines between her brows. As she put it, "I think I look mad all the time." Although this was something that concerned her, she didn't reveal it till our visit was almost over. This is remarkable but not uncommon. Many of my patients are embarrassed to mention what is really on their minds because they are afraid that I might think it is insignificant. Nothing is too insignificant to mention to your dermatologist. If it bothers you, speak up, because most of the time something can be done about it.

Doctor's Orders

It can be overwhelming to see the first real signs of aging change the landscape of your complexion, even in the tiniest ways. Sometimes it seems easier to ignore the signs entirely than to face your reflection, acknowledge what's happening, and seek treatment.

The mirror exercise that I used with Jessica is the best way for me to figure out which topicals or procedures will yield the results a particular patient wants. I encourage you to do the same exercise at home. Although it can be discouraging to view those lines and blotches front and center, the truth is far more encouraging: if you begin to battle the early signs of aging now, you could see significant improvement within a couple of months.

More and more often, people are looking to injectables to kick-start lowering their skin's virtual age. I treat nearly thirty patients a week with Botox, which gently relaxes the facial muscles and thus erases creases and lines on the upper face, around the mouth, and on the neck. My office calendar is also filled with the names of people who want to smooth away fine lines and deeper creases and replace lost volume in the face with injectable fillers. Hyaluronic acids, such as Restylane, Juvederm, and Perlane, are the most popular fillers, and collagens are still used somewhat, but newer formulas are entering the market all the time. Perhaps you've heard of some of the latest fillers, such as Sculptra and Radiesse.

Whether they are designed to relax wrinkles or to plump them, injectables are increasingly appealing, for three reasons. First, they offer instant gratification, or as close as you can get to it. (Fillers like Restylane and Juvederm fill the unwanted crease immediately, whereas Botox takes three days to start to work and ten days to take full effect.) Second, these treatments are relatively noninvasive and inexpensive, especially when you compare them to surgery; they require less than an hour of in-office time and cost far less than most people think they will. Third, since most injectables last for several months, it's hardly the end of the world if you're not wild about the outcome.

If the results don't fully meet your expectations, it's important to go back to see your physician. He or she might be able to correct or improve the job. It's also crucial for your doctor to see exactly what you don't like about the result so that he or she can make sure to modify the technique the next time. If, however, you're positive that you don't like your doctor's technique, seek out someone new next time.

Just remember that whether you're going under the needle for the first time or the tenth, it's imperative to keep your expectations in check. Injectable treatments can pick up where topicals leave off, providing a more aggressive way to knock years off the face, but they can't work miracles. Some signs of aging, like sun-induced brown spots, facial redness and broken vessels, diffuse textural changes, and sagging, might require lasers, light sources, peels, or (for pronounced sagging) even the scalpel to remedy.

This brings me to the most important point of all: even though "going under the syringe" comes with a minimal cost and time commitment, injectables are not treatments to take lightly. If you learn one thing from this chapter, let it be this: skip the Botox parties. When you see a billboard advertising cut-rate fillers at a spa that is not affiliated with a dermatologist you trust, keep driving.

Injecting these substances is a medical procedure and a true art form. The more careful you are about choosing an experienced dermatologist who is highly skilled and who approaches your treatment with artistry, the more likely you are to be thrilled with the results. Going to someone who is not artistically inclined, properly trained, or medically supervised can lead to, at best, a fake-looking outcome and, at worst, permanent damage to your face.

Now that we've gotten the caveats out of the way, let's take a more detailed look at the incredible injectables.

Botox

Patients like Jessica—women who never would have thought of using anything more than a nighttime facial cream on their faces just a year or so ago—are increasingly asking me about Botox. This is no surprise, considering how mainstream the treatment has become: you can't watch TV, read a beauty magazine, or go out to have drinks with your coworkers without the subject of Botox coming up. Nevertheless, many people are still a little scared of it. That's usually because they don't understand exactly what it is and how it works. I will address some of the questions I hear most often.

How does Botox work?

Botox is a neuromodulator that is produced by a type of bacterium called *Clostridium botulinum*, which is found virtually everywhere. By interfering with the nerve impulses that are responsible for muscular contractions, the toxin dramatically weakens or paralyzes certain muscles without causing any permanent damage. Its effects peak about ten days after injection and begin to gradually recede three to four months later. Botox works

Myth Some topical creams work just as well as Botox—without the needles.

Truth I can understand the temptation to choose a cream over Botox. The former is painless, available at the local drugstore, and less expensive than the muscle-weakening injectable—short-term, anyway. It's true that the right cream can tighten and firm the skin, and some peptide creams might subtly relax fine lines for several hours. However, even the best topicals simply don't compare to Botox, which actually stops those deep lines and creases from forming for four whole months, which means that it might actually be more cost-effective over the long run. A recent study compared Botox to several antiwrinkle creams, like StriVectin, and the results confirmed this.

best on the muscles that are involved in what dermatologists call the "lines of negative facial expression": the lines that form on your face when you feel sad, angry, or concerned. Botox is especially good at softening crow's feet as well as creases and wrinkles between the brows, above and below the lips, on the front of the neck, and across the forehead.

Isn't Botox a poison?

In large quantities, the bacteria used in Botox kill by paralyzing the muscles, so that breathing eventually stops. The doses we use to inject and weaken the tiny facial muscles that are responsible for creases and wrinkles are purified and very diluted, vastly lower than the levels considered toxic. We know this because Botox has been around since the late 1970s. For years doctors used it to treat muscle spasms of the eyes and neck. In 1997 the FDA approved it for the treatment of frown lines, and it's been used millions of times since then without any reports of allergic reactions or serious side effects, which is pretty remarkable.

Are there any side effects?

We administer Botox in a series of injections with very fine needles. These injections hurt, but done properly, they're barely painful and extremely well tolerated; any discomfort lasts only seconds. Temporary bruising is certainly possible. Treatments can occasionally lead to asymmetrical (or just plain odd-looking) results. Weakening the forehead muscles that control elevation can cause the brows to drop, causing you to look a bit like a caveman (or cavewoman). On the other hand, if those muscles are insufficiently weakened, you can wind up with too much elevation, making the outside edge of the brow just a bit too high and giving you a surprised look. When used around the eyebrows, Botox can inadvertently affect the eyelids, causing them to droop. If injected around the mouth improperly, the drug can overly weaken the lip muscles, forcing the lips to sag or making it hard for you to speak crisply, purse your lips, or kiss. If and when these side effects occur, they are usually short-lived, lasting a few days to a few weeks. Only occasionally do they last the full four months, until the Botox wears off.

All these scenarios are rare for those who go to an experienced injector: a dermatologist, a dermatological surgeon, or a plastic surgeon. Be sure to ask your doctor how long he or she has been treating patients with Botox and how many procedures he or she does per month. Also ask for the names of at least a few of the doctor's patients, so you can talk to them about their experiences. If your doctor seems at all threatened by your questions or you're uncomfortable with his or her responses, say thanks very much and leave. (Some states permit nurses to inject Botox. In the hands of a highly experienced nurse you should be fine, but I personally believe that you are much better off if a skilled dermatologist performs the treatment.)

On the positive side, even the most unsightly results last only four months, at the most. That's why, when my patients tell me that they wish Botox was permanent, I reply, "I'm not sure you would!" Frankly, if the results were permanent, Botox would never have been approved by the FDA as a treatment in the first place.

Botox injection sites

Glabellar muscles

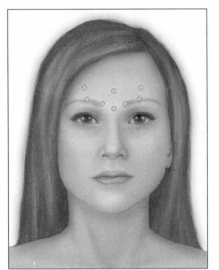 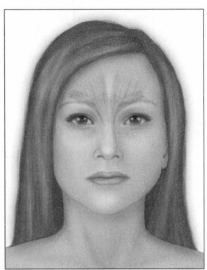

Botox sites on the forehead.

Doesn't Botox paralyze the face?

Of course it's *possible* to paralyze too many of the facial muscles and completely "freeze" the upper face. When Botox is done properly by an expert, however, this should not happen—that is, unless you want that sort of look. Our style is to make our patients look natural. It's the very rare person who *asks* me to make it so that his or her forehead doesn't move at all. I only have two patients for whom I'll actually do that—to achieve these results I use a much higher dose of Botox than I do for anyone else. They ask me, "Why would anyone do Botox and want their face to move even a little bit?" Meanwhile, some folks look at women like this and think, "Whoa, her forehead doesn't move. It looks like a plank of wood." Nevertheless, I comply. Beauty is in the eye of the beholder, and in these cases, as long as the patient is happy and likes the way she or he looks, we're not doing any harm.

Injecting is an art; a skilled dermatologist knows how to precisely calibrate the dose of Botox for each patient and customize the outcome to exactly what the patient wants. If she wants her eyebrows angled up a bit at the lateral edge or gently arched, we can do that. We can even elevate the entire brow. That's the difference between someone who injects with a lot of skill and experience and someone who's just okay at performing Botox treatments.

Does Botox always last four months?

The effect starts three days after injection and takes seven to ten days to reach its peak. The most noticeable results of Botox last for two months. During the third month, you'll feel a bit of movement in the treated area, and during the fourth month the effects drop off pretty quickly. We recommend re-treatment at about three and a half to four months, when the Botox is on its way out but not totally gone. It's sort of like getting your hair cut: it's best to do it just before you need it so that your hair looks nice all the time. (I'm sure you've had the experience of thinking it looks just fine one day and too long, too full, or just not right the next, and by then your stylist's calendar is packed.) Most of my patients book their next Botox treatment as they leave the office from the treatment we have just completed. This way they get a choice appointment time, and the interval between their treatments is just right. Others prefer to stretch out the time between visits for as long as possible and are very happy coming in for treatments as infrequently as twice a year. These patients wait till their Botox has pretty much worn off before they call to book their next treatment.

With regular injections, will my frown lines and creases eventually go away on their own?

Sorry, but no. However, some of my patients notice that after injecting on a regular basis every three and a half to four months for a while, they can eventually stretch out the interim time to four and a half months or even five months. The whole idea is to inject just often enough that the treated areas look nice and smooth all year long. You'll know that it's time for the next treatment when

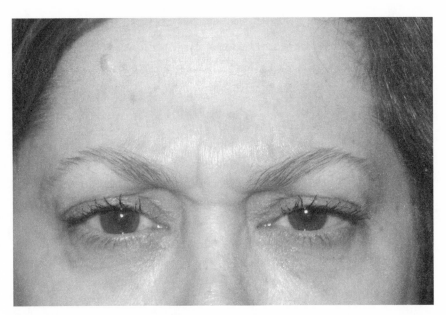

Before a Botox procedure for frown lines.

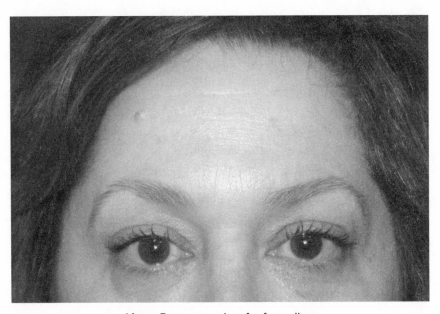

After a Botox procedure for frown lines.

your muscles have "recovered" from the last treatment and you're able to frown or crease the area. The creases should not be present when your face is at rest. (I do know a handful of patients who have trained themselves to stop frowning after using Botox for several years, but this is pretty uncommon.)

How old do you have to be to start Botox?

There's no set age. Many of us have noticed that starting before any lines have become ingrained seems to prevent permanent creasing of the skin. I'd venture to guess that if you begin Botox treatments early enough—possibly in your twenties or thirties— facial creases in the treated areas will most likely never form. On the other hand, there is nothing wrong with starting in your

Myth   Using Botox along with a filler is redundant and just a waste of money.

Truth   I'm going to let you in on a little secret—one that even some dermatologists don't know yet. A Botox-filler combination therapy is actually one of the most effective, underrated ways to erase and prevent fine lines, wrinkles, and deep folds. I still can't get over the spectacular results I saw after treating Dora, a fortysomething woman who came to see me last year. We started with a little Botox in her glabellar creases, the frown lines between the eyebrows. Although they faded a bit, the grooves had etched deeply into her skin, like pleats permanently ironed into a pair of pants. The moment I added a touch of the hyaluronic acid filler Restylane to those lines, however, they vanished.

The most miraculous part is this: a year later, all we've done is touch up with Botox every four months, with no additional filler, and we can't see one iota of the creases. It is clear that the two injectables work synergistically, each prolonging the life span of the other, with spectacular results. You spend more money up front, but the cash you save in the long run is well worth it. This two-pronged approach works especially well for anyone with deep frown lines between the brows. That includes men, whose creases tend to be even more stubborn and deeper that those of women. Of course, it usually takes the guy's wife to nudge him into my office!

forties, fifties, or even later. If the creases are relatively deep, keep in mind that it will take a few treatments for them to flatten out. If you've been frowning for twenty or thirty years, don't expect the creases to disappear a day or two after the first Botox treatment. Given time and a few visits, even the most stubborn deep creases respond.

When doctors say that starting Botox treatments early enough might stave off wrinkles and lines entirely, just how early do they mean?

I recently saw a twenty-seven-year-old patient who proves the power of thinking ahead. Molly was a really animated young woman who worked at Harvard University, not far from my office. Despite the fact that she was wearing no makeup, her skin was beautiful, except for a few horizontal forehead lines that I had to strain to see. Molly knew that they'd only get deeper with age, and a month earlier she had witnessed her sixty-year-old mother's face relax and become more youthful after just a few shots of Botox in her upper face and a bit of the cosmetic filler Restylane in her lower-face creases. "She looks great," Molly said. "Now I want to do some, but is it bad to start this early?" Not at all, I told her. In fact, we could also smooth the emerging nasolabial folds between the corners of her nose and her outer lips with the same Restylane her mom had used. After I finished up her filler injections, Molly was ecstatic and immediately booked her four-month follow-up appointment. Of course, it took a few days for the effects of her Botox treatment to show. When patients ask me whether they're too young for these treatments, I tell them to ignore their chronological age and look in the mirror. If they see issues that bug them, we'll take care of them. If they don't, we won't do anything, no matter their age.

What are the best places on the face to inject Botox?

We used to restrict Botox to the upper part of the face (frown lines, forehead creases, and crow's feet), but more recently we've started to treat other areas of the face, especially around the mouth and the neck, very successfully. A few examples of these newer treatment areas are "bunny" lines on the side of the nose, vertical lines around the upper and lower lips, dimpling on the chin, downturned corners of the mouth, and vertical bands on the neck. These areas, too, require treatment by a skilled expert with experience.

What about using Botox for excessive sweating?

Hyperhidrosis—a fancy term for excessive sweating—is an extremely common condition, especially in the underarms, palms, and soles. Now that more and more people are realizing how effective Botox is at treating it, increasing numbers of patients are asking for help. I've met people who spend their lives wearing only dark, heavy fabrics, shrouding themselves in two or three layers, simply to avoid the embarrassment of sweat soaking through their clothes. Those who are living with highly sweaty palms avoid shaking hands at all costs, which means they steer clear of most social situations. They even feel uncomfortable handling paper. The injectable works by blocking the nerves that stimulate perspiration, keeping the treated area completely dry for up to six months. The procedure, which is occasionally covered by insurance, is nearly pain-free for the underarms, but it can be quite uncomfortable for the palms and soles. It takes up to ten days until the area becomes totally dry, but once the effect kicks in, the treatment truly changes people's lives.

How much does Botox cost?

As with any other medical procedure, the price of Botox injections varies from city to city and doctor to doctor. The amount you'll pay depends on the amount of Botox used, how experienced your doctor is, and where in the country he or she practices. In general, treating the upper face can range between $500 and $1,000.

One of the most exciting things about Botox is that even

though the treatment has been around for decades and it's been approved by the FDA for cosmetic uses for more than ten years, we're still discovering new ways to use it. In addition to injecting it in the less conventional areas that I mentioned above (the sides of the nose, lip lines, chin dimples, vertical bands on the neck), some of us put minute amounts of Botox underneath the eyes to erase creases there, between the eyelids and the brows to achieve a slight but noticeable nonsurgical brow lift of a couple of millimeters, and at the outer corners of the eyes to open the eyes ever so slightly.

I've read about Botox alternatives—how do they compare?

Right now, we have only one other FDA-approved botulinum toxin at our disposal: Myobloc. It works, but it typically causes more discomfort than Botox does. Myobloc also costs more and doesn't last quite as long, so I can't think of any reason that a doctor would choose it over Botox. In Europe, a neuromodulator called Dysport—known in the United States as Reloxin—has been approved for years. It seems to work as well, and costs about the same, as Botox and could be approved by the FDA sometime in 2009. Doctors are also currently studying many more neuromodulators. None thus far appears to be significantly better than Botox. None appears to last that much longer or cost significantly less. Frankly, since Botox works so well and has so few side effects, it's hard to imagine that another substance would displace it anytime soon. Yet even though the next crop of neuromodulators that appear in doctors' offices might not offer patients significant new benefits, the competition can keep Botox prices from rising too high.

You can see why increasing numbers of people—even so-called low-maintenance folks—are making triannual Botox treatments a permanent part of their anti-aging arsenal. Still, let's face it: the wrinkle-relaxing drug can't do *everything.* Very deep glabellar creases and frown lines between the eyebrows will improve with Botox, but they often do not disappear completely, even after a series of injections spaced four months apart. Moreover, certain lines and wrinkles, especially those in the lower half of the face, don't respond to Botox at all. Remember that the treatment works by weakening the muscles and smoothing the lines that come from negative facial expressions: the expressions your face makes when you are angry, sad, or concerned. Botox is especially good at softening dynamic creases and wrinkles, such as the crease between the brows, horizontal creases across the forehead, crow's feet, vertical lines at the upper and lower lips, and bands that run down the front of the neck. Botox cannot soften static lines and crinkles that are present when your face is at rest. These are best smoothed out with fillers or with a laser or light source.

Deena's Story: The Miracle of Cosmetic Fillers

My other favorite injectable weapon is fillers. I was wrapping up a very busy week at the office recently when a new patient walked into my exam room. Deena was a blond, blue-eyed, fit, attractive woman who had spent her entire life riding horses. What surprised me most about her was her age. She told me she was fifty-seven, but she actually looked much older, surely because of her outdoor lifestyle. If she hadn't been diligent about wearing a high-SPF sunscreen every day, Deena would have looked even older. As it was, she had deep frown lines, horizontal grooves across her brow, and lines that ran from her nose to the outer corners of her mouth and then down to her chin. (We call those nasolabial folds and melolabial folds, respectively.)

Deena's husband had just gone away on a fishing trip to Mexico. Before he left, she had mentioned to him that she didn't like all the changes she was seeing in the mirror. While he was gone, she had vowed, she was going to do something about them. Naturally, Deena's husband had assured her that she already looked perfect and that he loved her just the way she was. These are comforting words, but Deena still came to see me as soon as he left town, wondering what she could possibly do to remedy the deepening wrinkles on her face.

"If you'd like, we can do a little something today," I told her. I explained that Botox would do wonders for the frown lines, the creases on her forehead, and the crow's feet, and that it would soften the vertical bands of her neck. For the nasolabial and melolabial lines, however, I suggested Restylane, which is made of hyaluronic acid, a spongy, water-absorbing substance that the body produces just beneath the skin. Best of all, I added, the filler's effects would be immediate. I could tell by her face that she was both petrified and very excited. Timidly, she answered, "Why don't we give it a try?" Deena found the Botox injections fairly easy to take, but she found the Restylane injections rather uncomfortable. We coached her through the process, and the pain went away the moment I removed the needle. Ten minutes later she was smiling into the mirror, repeating, "I can't believe they're gone." Deena's lines weren't really completely gone, but they had improved 70 to 80 percent that afternoon. She was ecstatic, and she agreed that the results were well worth the discomfort. "I'm so glad I ignored my husband," she joked as she left the office.

Deena is a remarkably down-to-earth woman; there's nothing fancy or high-maintenance about her. She has a no-makeup lifestyle and simply wanted, like so many of us, to wake up every morning without looking progressively older. There's certainly no shame in that, especially now that fillers are so simple and affordable to obtain. Botox and Restylane were great choices for Deena, not only because the spongy gel smoothed her creases so naturally and effectively but also because it's one filler that requires no allergy testing. This meant that we could begin the injections immediately, before she could scare herself into never coming back and before her friends or her husband could talk her out of it. After just one appointment, Deena looked years younger. She won't have to return for Botox for another four months, and she can wait six months for her next treatment with Restylane.

Cosmetic Fillers

As fillers become more widely available and as dermatologists become increasingly adept at using them, it's easy to take stories like Deena's for granted. A few injections here, a few injections there, and voilà! she's taken years off her face. However, the injectable-filler field is relatively young and has only recently grown by leaps and bounds.

Let's define what fillers actually are. In short, they do just what they say: they fill unwanted folds, creases, and wrinkles in the skin. Some are for small and shallow superficial creases, others are for deeper folds, and some of the newest ones are specifically designed to address the volume loss that occurs naturally with aging and that usually leads to the drooping and sagging we associate with our grandparents' faces.

From the late 1970s until 2002, bovine collagen (collagen from cows) was the first and only filler approved by the Food and Drug Administration for use in the United States. Sold under the names Zyderm and Zyplast, it wasn't hugely popular and didn't get a great deal of press because it wasn't a great filler. Doctors used it primarily to plump up the edges of the lips and to smooth nasolabial and melolabial folds. Because the collagen was derived from cattle (a special herd that is raised and cared for specifically for collagen production), about 3 percent of patients were allergic to the material. This meant that we had to perform two skin tests four weeks apart to ensure that the individual wasn't allergic before we could proceed with the treatment. Because of the minimum six-week wait between the day a patient expressed interest in the filler and the day it was injected, many people would change their minds. For those who stayed the course, the results lasted only three to four months, at the very most.

For thirty years, dermatologists had only that *one* type of filler available, which is pretty remarkable, considering what came next. Human collagen (Cosmoderm and Cosmoplast), which won approval early in 2003, represented a huge advance over the bovine formula. It worked at least as well, but since it didn't cause allergic reactions, it didn't require tedious skin tests. You could decide you wanted your lips plumped up one minute and view the results in the mirror ten minutes later.

That's when the injectable-filler field truly took off. In the late 1990s, a brilliant Swedish doctor posed the question that no one

What's in a Name?

One of the reasons the cosmetic-filler field can be confusing is that it's called by so many different names. Some dermatologists refer to these substances mainly by their generic labels, like collagen and hyaluronic acid. Most of them prefer to use brand names, such as Cosmoplast, Restylane, and Juvederm. The majority probably use brand names and generic names interchangeably. Perhaps this handy reference guide will help you to keep the labels straight.

Generic name: bovine collagen
Brand names: Zyderm and Zyplast

Generic name: human collagen
Brand names: Cosmoderm and Cosmoplast

Generic name: hyaluronic acid
Brand names: Restylane, Perlane, Juvederm Ultra, Juvederm Ultra Plus, Hylaform, Prevelle Silk, Captique, and Puragen

Generic name: poly-L-lactic acid (PLLA)
Brand name: Sculptra

Generic name: calcium hydroxylapatite
Brand name: Radiesse

Generic name: polymethyl methacrylate (PMMA) beads embedded in collagen
Brand name: ArteFill

Generic name: porcine collagen (collagen from pigs)
Brand name: Evolence

seemed to be asking: Why are we injecting collagen into the face when we could be using hyaluronic acid, the spongy, thick gel in our skin that supports the body's own collagen fibers? The FDA approved the first hyaluronic acid filler (Restylane) in December 2003. The allergic reaction rate was very low, so no skin tests were necessary, and doctors and patients loved the fact that Restylane lasted an average of six months, compared to collagen's two- to four-month life span. Furthermore, the results were very natural looking, and the filler was extremely versatile; it was just as good at filling lips as it was at smoothing nasolabial and melolabial folds and forehead frown lines. No wonder the substance became so popular almost immediately after it hit the market. It has overtaken collagen as a filler in popularity ever since.

Now that it's possible to immediately plump up creases, folds, lips, and hollow areas, with incredibly natural-looking results, the awareness of and interest in fillers has increased tremendously throughout the country. (They're no longer reserved for eccentric, fake-looking actresses and socialites.) Ever since Restylane's approval, other manufacturers have been trying to catch up. I have many hyaluronic acid injectables at my disposal, including Juvederm Ultra and Juvederm Ultra Plus, as well as Perlane, which appears to work at least as nicely as Restylane. It's certainly nice to have options, and those options continue to expand as longer-lasting fillers like Sculptra, Radiesse, and other substances continue to be developed.

Volume Fillers

If you have the chance to study a child's face, you'll probably notice that his or her youthful look comes largely from full lips, big eyes, and plump, round cheeks. As we move through adulthood, our face shape lengthens. Our eyes begin to look smaller, and our lips become thinner. Deep creases might eventually form, especially around the nose, mouth, and chin, and break up the contour of the face,

Only later does everything start to sag. Fat redistribution is common with aging. We lose fat in our cheeks, and it accumulates under our chin and as puffiness under our eyes. Think of a relative who has recently dropped a couple of sizes; although she looks great, for the most part, you can't get over the fact that her face looks a little more severe, a little older. Consider the attractive friend who is a bit under his ideal body weight. He used to look fabulous, but with age, his face appears too thin and makes him seem suddenly older. (I know people who are actually afraid to lose ten or fifteen pounds because of this.) That's where volume fillers come in. Injected properly, they fill hollow cheeks and produce immediate improvement—instant youth.

There's no doubt about it: fillers work. The question is how do you know which ones will work for *you*? When I consulted with Deena, we considered her lifestyle and age, examined exactly *how* her skin was aging, then worked together to determine the ideal treatment for her. Given the myriad of choices of fillers, it's easy to feel bewildered when you're trying to choose what's best for you. Pinpointing the perfect option starts with visiting a doctor you trust, someone with extensive experience injecting many different kinds of fillers. You should have the opportunity to meet, or at least speak, with some of his or her patients. Your dermatologist should be able to clearly explain how each filler varies from the others and then discuss the risks and benefits of each, how long each one lasts, and which one suits you best.

Myth   The longer the filler lasts, the better it is.

Truth   Long-lasting and permanent fillers, like fat, Sculptra, Radiesse, and silicone are great because they require fewer follow-up visits (not to mention needles sticking you) to maintain your beautiful results. Unfortunately, not everyone sees the results that he or she desires, and the longer a filler's life span, the longer you have to put up with those unsatisfactory results. This means that permanent fillers can have permanent side effects. If your doctor overdoes it on your lips or fills your cheeks unevenly, or if you develop an allergic reaction, it can be difficult, time-consuming, and often impossible to remove the substance. In general, I discourage patients who have never used a filler before from using a long-lasting filler. Always start with a shorter–life span filler, such as one of the hyaluronic acids. If you like the results, you can always move on to a material with more longevity.

Many of my patients ask me about the likelihood of allergic reaction. "Doctor," they say, "if we're injecting a foreign substance under my skin, how do I know I won't wind up with unsightly lumps, blotches, or something worse?" It's a smart question. The truth is that you just don't know which substances you'll be sensitive to until they actually get under your skin, so buyer beware. Allergic reactions occasionally emerge immediately after a collagen treatment, but more often they show up about four weeks later, appearing as mild red swelling at the injection site. Generally, the reaction is painless but embarrassing. We treat these kinds of reactions with an immune-altering cream called Protopic, then let the bumps slowly but surely disappear on their own.

Fortunately, however, allergic reactions to the new fillers are rare. When such reactions do occur, they're usually mild and short-lived. The reason we don't require skin tests with hyaluronic acid injectables is that even though the substance is derived in a laboratory from either streptococcus bacteria or a rooster's comb, it's very pure and totally sterile by the time it is put into the syringe. Furthermore, it's engineered to be identical to, or very close to, the hyaluronic acid that our own bodies make. Immediately after a hyaluronic acid filler injection, most patients have a bit of redness that lasts a few hours and swelling that can last for a day or two. These reactions are most common with Restylane and Perlane, but the typical redness and inflammation don't constitute an allergic reaction. True allergic reactions are very uncommon.

In rare cases, about four weeks after injection, patients develop a bit of red swelling at the site of the injection. Like the allergic reactions to collagen, these bumps don't hurt, but they don't look good either. These, too, will go away on their own, but we can speed up their disappearance either by applying Protopic cream or by injecting an enzyme called hyaluronidase, which helps to break up the hyaluronic acid so that the injected material disappears from your skin. If this reaction happens to you, keep in mind that there's a chance you can still tolerate other hyaluronic acid fillers. For instance, if Restylane doesn't agree with you, you might do absolutely fine with Juvederm. Your doctor should be able to coach you through your options.

If you would like to try a filler but are a highly allergic person and are afraid you might react to it, I'd suggest that you start with a skin test. Your doctor will simply inject a small amount of the filler into your forearm. If after four to six weeks you don't see swelling, redness, blisters, or scabs, you're ready to have the filler injected into the desired crease. Just keep in mind that finding your ideal filler is sometimes an exercise in trial and error.

I vividly remember the first time I treated one of my favorite patients. Chic and elegant, Phoebe was a stylish sixty-year-old woman with spiked hair set off by funky multicolored tints. She had come to hate the lumps and lines that had developed along her upper lip, so I suggested filling them with bovine collagen. Both of her skin tests came out negative, yet Phoebe woke up four weeks later to find that the area we had injected had become red and swollen. We treated her with Protopic cream, which subdued the reaction gradually, over a few months.

Phoebe was delighted to be rid of the redness and the swelling, but she still had those upper-lip lines. We decided to treat them with the recently approved hyaluronic acid filler Hylaform after testing it first on her forearm. Phoebe's lip lines disappeared (with no allergic reaction) just in time for her daughter's wedding. More recently, we've moved on to Juvederm, the most recently approved hyaluronic acid filler, because it lasts twice as long as Hylaform. The results have been even more stunning. Phoebe is thrilled, and so am I.

If you're not sure which filler is best for which area, here are some tips on where each substance works best:

- Filling the lips makes the mouth look softer and less wrinkled and makes the entire face look younger.

- The right filler helps to smooth the vertical lines that form above the lips during the forties, fifties, and sixties. Shallow short lines are easier to erase than deeper, sharper ones.

- Botox can erase crow's feet, open the eyes, and raise the eyebrows without surgery. Adding a soft filler under the eyebrows and into the tails of the brows lifts them slightly, making the eyes look more open.

- Nasolabial folds, which extend from the outer nostrils to the corners of the lips, and melolabial folds, which run from the corners of the lips to the chin, break up the lower half of the face, making it appear much older. Injecting the right filler softens them.
- Botox is the treatment of choice for deep frown lines. If the lines are very deep, adding a filler can help enormously and can also help to preserve a Botox treatment's life span.
- In some cases, the eyes tend to gain fat, and surgery is the best solution. In other cases, the eyes lose fat with age, making the area appear sunken and exaggerating shadows and dark circles. Using the right filler in the tear trough (the sunken area just beneath the inner corners of the eyes) can all but erase those shadows, creating a younger, well-rested look.

How Fillers Work

I can vividly remember the day I met Sharon, a fifty-year-old woman who is now a regular patient in my office. When I introduced myself, she smiled, shook my hand, and got right down to business. She was troubled by her increasingly hollow cheeks and, after exhaustive research, decided that she was ready to replace the lost volume with a filler like Sculptra or Radiesse. It is so refreshing to meet with well-informed patients. Having a solid idea of what you want—your options, the relative risks and rewards, how much time and money you're willing to spend—before you see the doctor will help both of you to make an educated decision about the type of treatment that's right for you.

This does not mean that I expect my patients to plow through dry dermatology journals or spend hours a week surfing medical Web sites. I've created a summary of the most basic, relevant information for the substances that are available now, so that you're well armed if you do decide to have a cosmetic-filler conversation with your doctor. Notice that I said the fillers that are available *now*—at press time and in this country. Keep in mind that the landscape is constantly evolving. Right now, more than fifty fillers are available in Europe that aren't approved in the United States. The best ones will wind up making it to this side of the Atlantic, but many more will not.

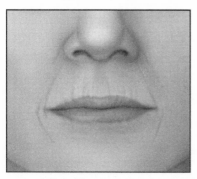

Before fillers are injected

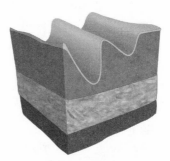

Cross section of the skin
before filling

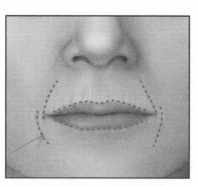

Filler is placed in each of the areas
shown by the dotted line

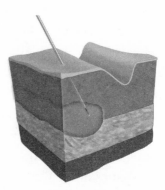

One wrinkle filled

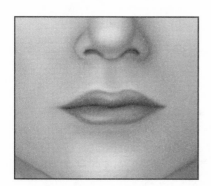

After fillers are injected

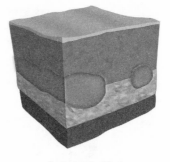

Completely filled

Filler injection: before and after.

Each filler requires a different technique on the dermatologist's part, and it is ideal if your doctor is familiar and comfortable with several formulas. I certainly have my favorite fillers, but we have all of the available ones in my office. This worked out well for Sharon. We ended up replacing lost volume in her cheeks with Sculptra, but we could just as easily have used Radiesse, the other great volume filler that she mentioned.

In my office we often use several different kinds of cosmetic fillers on one patient to produce the best results. For example, for deep nasolabial or melolabial folds, we sometimes inject a thicker filler below, such as Perlane or Juvederm Ultra Plus, and a thinner or softer one above, such as Restylane or Juvederm Ultra, layering them on top of each other. Then for the hollows of the cheek we might use either Radiesse or Sculptra.

Working with cosmetic fillers is truly an art form. It's a little like painting a portrait or a landscape. Few great artists rely on only one color or texture. They vary their shades and alter the thickness of the paint to achieve their desired effect. So when you are searching for a dermatologist, resist the urge to look for the least expensive deal or the closest doctor's office. Choose someone who views your skin as a palette and is a true master at his or her craft. After all, you have only one face. The idea is to walk out looking natural and beautiful, not filled.

Myth Substances and treatments that are used off-label are dangerous; it's best to stay away from them.

Truth The term *off-label* simply means that the substance has been approved by the FDA only for a use other than the one you're considering. For instance, silicone is approved for a certain type of eye-injection procedure, but dermatologists' use of it as a cosmetic filler is off-label unless or until a company submits the necessary data to prove that it's safe to use in that capacity. In other words, off-label treatments aren't necessarily unsafe; the safety and effectiveness data for that particular purpose have not been submitted to the FDA.

Types of Fillers

There are many types of fillers on the market today. Some are better suited for one part of the face than others. This list categorizes some of the more popular fillers along with their pros and cons. You and your doctor can decide which of these is best for the areas you want to treat.

Zyderm and Zyplast (Bovine Collagen)

What it is. Zyderm and Zyplast are made from collagen that is derived from a herd of cattle raised specifically for this purpose. Zyderm is the softer, more malleable, and shorter lasting of the two fillers, whereas Zyplast is firmer and has a longer life span.

What it's best for. Zyderm is best for fine lines around the lips, fine lines elsewhere on the face, and glabellar creases. Zyplast works beautifully in the body of the lips, in deeper lines such as the nasolabial and melolabial folds, and in other deep creases around the chin and the cheeks.

How long it lasts. Zyderm lasts two months, whereas Zyplast lasts three to four months.

Pros. Since both fillers flow smoothly from the syringe, they deliver a beautiful, natural look. Patients typically see very little swelling after injection, so in most instances you can be treated in the afternoon and safely go out in public that evening.

Cons. Because Zyderm and Zyplast come from cattle and contain animal proteins, they cause allergic reactions in about 3 percent of the people injected with it. Two skin tests that are done four weeks apart are essential before treatment. Occasionally, even those who have two negative skin tests will have an allergic reaction to the treatment. Collagen's short life span means that you have to return frequently to maintain the results.

Cosmoderm and Cosmoplast (Human Collagen)

What it is. Cosmodern and Cosmoplast are collagen that is derived from human baby foreskin cells that have been cultured in a lab. Cosmoderm is the softer, more malleable, shorter-lasting of the two, whereas Cosmoplast is firmer and lasts longer.

What it's best for. We use Cosmoderm like Zyderm, to smooth fine lines on the upper lip, fine lines elsewhere on the face, and glabellar creases. Cosmoplast is used like Zyplast. It's better suited for the body of the lip, deeper lines such as the nasolabial and melolabial folds, and other deep creases of the chin and the cheeks.

How long it lasts. Cosmoderm lasts two months, whereas Cosmoplast lasts three to four months.

Pros. Because these products are made from human cells, there's very little risk of allergic reaction, which means that no skin test is required. Both formulas flow easily from the syringe, leaving a naturally beautiful look. As with Zyderm and Zyplast, you can generally go out in public a few hours after treatment, since postinjection swelling is quite minimal.

Cons. Collagen's short life span means that you have to return frequently to maintain the results.

Restylane, Perlane, Juvederm Ultra and Juvederm Ultra Plus, Hylaform, Prevelle Silk, Captique, and Puragen (Hyaluronic Acid)

What it is. This category of products is a bioengineered version of the spongy, water-absorbent material produced by the body that helps to hold collagen and elastin together, giving the skin support and body. Restylane and Perlane are derived from the streptococcus bacteria, whereas Hylaform and Juvederm come from roosters' combs.

What it's best for. These extremely versatile fillers are useful for the nasolabial and melolabial folds, glabellar creases, and smile lines. They can also fill the lips, the cheeks, and the tear trough.

How long it lasts. These products last six months or more.

Pros. There's very little risk of allergic reaction, which means that no skin test is required and your dermatologist can inject on the spot. The hyaluronic acid fillers are versatile and produce very natural-looking results.

Cons. Postinjection swelling from Restylane and Perlane, which is especially noticeable after treating the lips, lasts a day or two. Swelling after Juvederm treatments is less dramatic. Allergic reactions are possible but rare.

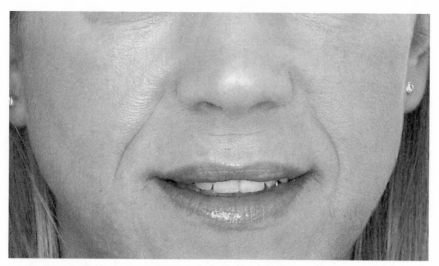

Before Restylane treatment.

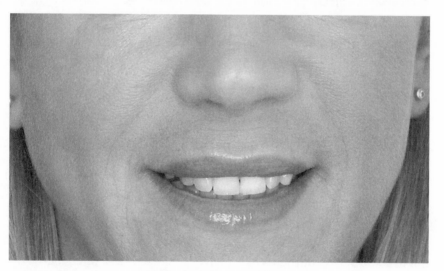

After Restylane treatment.

Fat

What it is. Your body's own fat can also be used as a filler. During a minor operation that is performed under local anesthesia and that leaves only a tiny mark behind, your doctor removes portions of unwanted fat from places like the belly or the neck. After cleansing and sterilizing the fat, he or she injects it into anesthetized areas on the face that require volume filling.

What it's best for. Fat is used for facial recontouring and adding volume, especially in the nasolabial folds and cheeks.

How long it lasts. Fat injections last more than a year.

Pros. Fat is versatile, and since it comes from your own body, it's the ultimate natural filler. Furthermore, most of us have an abundant supply, so the fat itself costs nothing. Finally, since it can be harvested in advance and kept for eighteen months in a medical freezer, your doctor can easily provide touch-ups during the year and a half after the first treatment.

Cons. Although the fat itself is free, the procedure to remove and prepare it is complicated and thus more expensive than using an engineered filler. Injections require a large needle, which means that treatments are painful (and require anesthesia) and usually lead to swelling and bruising that lasts several days. Fat is not good for the lips; it makes them look like pillows.

Sculptra (Poly-L-lactic Acid)

What it is. Sculptra is made from poly-L-lactic acid, a synthetic powder that is derived from absorbable suture material. It's used as a volume filler for facial contouring and to fill deep lines, hollows, and depressions. Before we inject it, we mix the powder with sterile water and a bit of local anesthetic, then let it sit for a few hours—or even better, a few days. Sculptra works differently from most other fillers: it stimulates your own body to produce collagen. That means you might look beautiful the day you have it injected, but once the water is absorbed and the temporary plumping goes away, you'll look pretty much the way you did before for quite a while. Generally you need a minimum of three treatments, one month apart, to see lasting results. With each subsequent treatment, your skin produces more and more collagen. At press time, Sculptra was approved by the FDA only for facial atrophy in HIV patients. Nevertheless, doctors are currently using it off-label for many other cosmetic purposes, and studies are under way for FDA approval for those uses.

What it's best for. Sculptra is best for filling volume loss anywhere in the face, including the cheeks, the nasolabial and melolabial folds, and under and around the eyes.

How long it lasts. Sculptra lasts at least one year and possibly as long as three years.

Pros. Sculptra is long lasting, natural looking, and versatile, filling deep spaces and hollows as well as deep lines.

Cons. Since Sculptra works by stimulating collagen production, you won't see any improvement until you've had at least a few treatments. Injections are painful and usually require anesthesia. You'll also notice some swelling and bruising after each treatment. Sculptra is not a good filler for the lips.

Radiesse (Calcium Hydroxylapatite)

What it is. Radiesse is a very thick, almost pasty, white material that contains spheres made from a synthetic version of the material found in bones and teeth. It has been used for years to heal damaged vocal cords and other tissue. Once the spheres are injected, the body slowly produces collagen around them.

What it's best for. Radiesse is a volume filler that works best for deep nasolabial and melolabial folds and for hollow cheeks. It is not suited for the lips. Swelling and bruising that last a few days after treatment are common.

How long it lasts. The biggest advantage of Radiesse is how long it lasts, which is from one year to eighteen months. (We occasionally recommend a touch-up treatment a few weeks after the first session, however.)

Pros. Because the results of Radiesse last a year or more, you need fewer follow-up treatments to maintain your look. Thus, even though Radiesse costs more per treatment than some other fillers, the expense balances out in the long run.

Cons. Radiesse is thicker than collagen, Restylane, or Juvederm Ultra, so a bigger needle is required to inject it. That means that the risk of bruising and swelling, which last for a few days, is higher than with other fillers. The treatments are painful, which means that you'll probably be given a topical anesthetic like Xylocaine first. Radiesse is not suited for the lips.

ArteFill

What it is. ArteFill is made from microspheres of polymethyl methacrylate (or Lucite) that are suspended in bovine collagen. The collagen is absorbed by the body in two to four months, leaving behind tiny spherical beads of Lucite, which last forever. That makes ArteFill a truly permanent filler. Most doctors perform two or three treatments to ensure that all the creases are filled completely but subtly.

What it's best for. ArteFill is best for deep wrinkles, including nasolabial and melolabial folds and cheek creases.

How long it lasts. ArteFill lasts forever. However, as you age, the creases that you've filled might deepen, so you might require a touch-up two or more years after your initial series of treatments.

Pros. ArteFill is a permanent filler.

Cons. Permanent fillers have permanent complications. Because ArteFill lasts (and lasts), there's not much you can do if you don't like the results, so talk with your doctor to be sure it's right for you before getting started. The news is worse if you happen to be allergic to the material, because it can be very difficult to remove. Since the Lucite beads are embedded in bovine collagen, you must undergo two skin tests before embarking on treatment. ArteFill should not be used for the lips.

Liquid Injectable Silicone

What it is. One of the only truly permanent fillers available, silicone is a type of polymer that comes as a liquid-, oil-, or gel-based structure. It is clear, colorless, tasteless, thick, and viscous. In order to be considered injectable-grade (or medical-grade) silicone, the material must be filtered, purified, and sterilized. Like Sculptra, silicone is injected in microdroplet form into the middle skin layer, where it stimulates collagen production. Slowly but surely, over a series of four to six treatments, collagen builds up to fill the crease, fold, or hollow, leaving a pleasing and natural look.

What it's best for. Although it's not approved by the FDA as a cosmetic skin filler, silicone *is* approved for injection into the eye for treating a detached retina. Dermatologists use it off-label for moderate to deep lines, folds, and creases, such as nasolabial and melolabial folds. We also inject it into the lips, into cheek hollows, and into depressed scarring from acne and chicken pox.

How long it lasts. Silicone lasts forever. However, as you age, the creases that you've filled might deepen, so you might require a touch-up two or more years after your initial series of treatments.

Pros. Silicone is incredibly versatile, natural looking, permanent, and less expensive than other fillers.

Cons. The biggest con is that silicone lasts forever. If you don't ensure that you're getting purified, medical-grade silicone, you might react adversely to the foreign material that is mixed into it. As with all fillers, treatment success is based on your doctor's skill. If your dermatologist hasn't mastered the microdroplet technique, there's a good chance that he or she will inject more silicone than necessary, possibly leading to lumps.

Evolence

One of the very latest fillers that dermatologists are buzzing over is Evolence, a collagen that is derived from pigs. Why do we need another collagen filler? The big lure is that Evolence lasts longer than the traditional versions, possibly as long as one year. It mimics the body's own collagen, breaking down slowly and naturally over time. Furthermore, the manufacturers have developed different forms: a fine, softer type that is ideal for the tear trough and for glabellar creases and a firmer type for the lips and for nasolabial and melolabial folds. There's even a firm, bigger-particle type for volume filling. Evolence was recently approved by the FDA for use in the United States.

Tracy's Story: The Eyes Have It

By now, most people know that fillers can do wonders for fine lines around the eyes and the mouth, for creases between the brows, and for lips that have begun to thin. Few, however, even consider that these substances can do anything about the dark under-eye circles that become more pronounced as we get older. These circles emerge for a variety of reasons, but one of the most common is that the area around the eyes loses fat and volume with age. Tracy, a longtime patient of mine, can attest to that. When she was forty, her friends and coworkers began to tell her that she looked tired all the time. In fact, Tracy got plenty of sleep most nights and was well rested. She wanted to look as good as she felt.

When she asked for my opinion last year, I pointed out that the receding fat was making her eyes look hollow and was accentuating the shadows in the tear trough. Eyelid surgery really wasn't an option for Tracy, because she didn't have excess fat or skin to remove. Pulling the existing skin tighter would only make her look more severe. Instead, we tried a far less aggressive approach right in my office. We injected the crease just under her eyes with a hyaluronic acid filler, which made her eyes look more lively and her under-eye bags less noticeable. Although we didn't technically lighten the skin at all, we made the area *seem* brighter by taking away the shadowy hollow spots.

I performed the injections incredibly gently, so Tracy didn't require any anesthetic. Even though she experienced a tiny bit of swelling, which went away in a day or two, she had no bruising. Since I like to inject very conservative amounts, I suggested that she come back for a touch-up two weeks later if she thought the area required more volume. However, Tracy was extremely happy. The results lasted about six months, at which point we refilled the tear trough.

8

Lasers and Light Options

L asers are probably the most exciting class of devices that I have in my office. That's because they have the power to help my patients in so many ways: smoothing away fine lines and wrinkles, erasing decades' worth of brown spots, tightening sagging skin, and banishing unwanted hair—all within minutes, usually with very little recovery time. For many people, however, including some doctors, lasers and light sources remain shrouded in mystery. This chapter should dispel some of the confusion. Once again, before you start reading, I'd like you to take this quiz to see how savvy you already are about these powerful devices.

1. Laser treatments involve considerable pain and weeks of recovery
   A. All the time
   B. Sometimes
   C. Rarely

2. In terms of smoothing fine lines and sun-induced brown spots, how do lasers compare to prescription retinoids?

   A. They're far more powerful and achieve more dramatic results.

   B. The two treatments offer comparable results.

   C. Retinoids are more effective.

3. If I decide to treat my skin with a laser or a light source, how predictable are the results?

   A. It depends on the problem I'm treating and which device my doctor uses.

   B. Highly predictable. These treatments have come a long way and typically achieve great results.

   C. Always unpredictable. Regardless of the device that is used, there's no way for my doctor to estimate what the results will look like.

4. Laser treatments can _____ facial red blood vessels.

   A. do very little for. My best bet is to use a topical anti-redness cream.

   B. cure. They work so well that the vessels never return.

   C. clear. They won't stop new ones from developing, however.

5. Laser hair removal is a very effective treatment for nearly everyone, except

   A. Those with blond or white hair

   B. Those with dark skin

   C. Those with very dark hair

6. Thermage and other skin-tightening treatments are best for firming up the following:

   A. Facial areas like the jaw, chin, and eyelids

   B. The inner thighs and upper arms

   C. A wrinkly belly

   D. All of the above

7. What is the best method for banishing the majority of visible veins?

   A. Sclerotherapy

   B. Lasers and light sources

   C. Surgery

8. Cellulite creams are very effective under what condition?

   A. I'm willing to spend a lot of cash on them.

   B. I buy one designed by a dermatologist.

   C. These creams rarely result in much improvement.

9. Mesotherapy is

   A. A laser treatment designed to reduce cellulite

   B. A very questionable treatment that involves injecting detergents and other ingredients that supposedly melt away fat

   C. A specialized massage that smoothes away dimples and puckers

10. Dermatologic lasers expose the skin to light that is

    A. Dangerous when used more than once per year in the same area

    B. So gentle that I can comfortably book a treatment anywhere, including my neighborhood spa

    C. Usually very safe, as long as they're administered properly by a dermatologist, a plastic surgeon, or a provider supervised by one of these specialists

Answers

1. B: Many patients associate all laser treatments with raw, crusty skin and long postoperative periods that involve hiding out in a dark room. A few of the most aggressive treatments do cause pain and require downtime, but most of the treatments we use are brief procedures that are minimally uncomfortable and that heal very quickly, usually in a few hours to a couple of days.

2. A: I'm a huge fan of prescription topical retinoids, but if you want instant improvement, lasers and light sources are the way to go. Of course, the best way to keep your skin in top shape is to use a combination of retinoid creams and more aggressive treatments like lasers, though not at the same time.

3. B: Most of the new advanced lasers and light systems, like the powerful Q-switched lasers, fractional devices, and intense pulsed-light devices, offer predictably excellent results.

4. C: Lasers can reduce the facial redness and the visible blood vessels often associated with rosacea by as much as 90 percent. The treatment is not a permanent cure, however. New vessels will form in people who are prone to them, but you can keep them partly at bay by avoiding exposure to the sun, extreme temperatures, and certain foods.

5. A: Laser hair removal has always been ideal for people with very dark hair and pale skin. I'm happy to say that we now have devices that also work quite well on dark skin. Blond and white hair is still a challenge, though. It's often best removed by more conventional methods.

6. D: Tightening devices like Thermage, Titan, and ReFirme now come with a range of hand pieces in various sizes that allow us to firm very small areas on the face (a sagging jawline, chin, or eyelids) as well as larger off-face spots such as the belly, the thighs, and the upper arms.

7. A: Lasers are wonderful inventions, but tried-and-true sclerotherapy remains the gold standard for taking care of most veins. Read on for more about this popular, very effective treatment.

8. C: I'm sorry to say that even though some cellulite creams might make the dimpling less noticeable for a short time, I've never seen any data that prove that any of these formulas actually make the condition go away.

9. B: This procedure, which is *not* approved by the FDA, involves the injection of ingredients purported to melt away fat. I tell my patients to avoid the treatment until I find well-done scientific studies that prove its safety and effectiveness.

10. C: Lasers have been around for decades. All use rays of light that come from the milder visible and infrared portion of the light spectrum—the light that doesn't cause mutations linked to cancer. The fact remains, however, that lasers work by causing a controlled injury to the skin. Thus, it's imperative that you choose a practitioner who has a lot of experience, preferably a doctor or someone supervised by a doctor.

Myth   Lasers and energy-source devices expose the skin to dangerous forms of light.

Truth   Lasers have been around since the early 1960s, so if they emitted dangerous, cancer-causing forms of light, we'd know it by now. Many people associate these treatments with X-rays, which can strip electrons from the molecules in the body, inducing mutations that can turn into cancer over time. The light sources used in lasers and intense pulsed light come, for the most part, from the milder *visible light* portion of the spectrum. That means that these devices cannot strip electrons or cause the mutations that are linked to cancer.

Gail's Story: How Lasers Work

"I don't want a laser treatment—I've read that they burn the skin and leave it covered in scabs." I used to hear this all the time from my patients, many of whom assumed that all lasers were created equal. They also believed that every laser procedure resulted in raw, crusty skin and several weeks of recovery. This is not true anymore. Times have really changed.

I took care of a lovely couple: Gail, who was in her late forties, and her husband, Henry, who was in his early fifties. They came to my office together—although, as is often the case with couples, only she was interested in treatment at first. A former sun addict, she had become increasingly concerned with the hundreds of brown spots (lentigines, in dermatology-speak) that speckled her face, legs, and arms. A highly intelligent, stylish woman, Gail was a trendsetter and a fashion buyer for a high-end clothing company based in Rhode Island who frequently traveled to New York City on buying trips. Suddenly, she felt a lot of pressure to look as young and polished as possible. Nevertheless, when I suggested removing her spots with a Q-switched laser, she shuddered. "I don't have time to sit in the house while my skin heals," Gail said, adding that, frankly, she had a very low threshold for pain.

Gail wasn't entirely wrong in her concerns. It's true that a few laser treatments, like the powerful CO_2 resurfacing laser, work essentially by

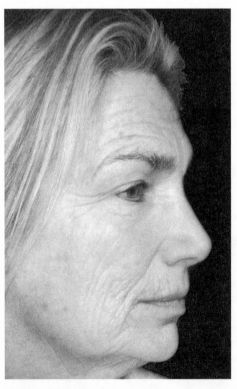

Before CO_2 laser skin resurfacing treatment.

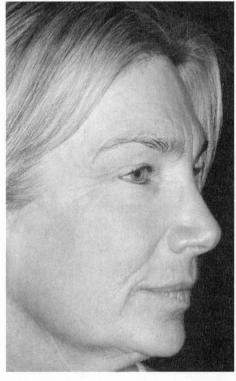

After CO_2 laser skin resurfacing treatment.

burning off the uppermost layers of the skin. Although a single treatment will eventually make your complexion look dramatically better—and lower your SVA considerably—you have to suffer through two to three weeks of recovery before you're ready to face the world. However, this type of aggressive laser treatment is the exception rather than the rule. There are many other lasers that come with little or no downtime. Some are so gentle that we use them to remove port-wine stain (i.e., reddish-purple colored) birthmarks on newborn babies.

If this seems hard to believe, consider the following analogy, which I use to reassure patients about lasers: You probably own a car that you use to drive to work or to run errands. Perhaps your children ride a large, lumbering bus to school or to field trips. Both vehicles have wheels and seats. Both run on gasoline. Yet it would be just as silly to use a bus for a family grocery-shopping run as it would be to use a car to transport forty students on a school trip. In other words, even though each vehicle falls in the category of transportation, each serves its own distinct purpose.

The same goes for lasers. By definition, all of them affect the skin in a localized area through a powerful beam of light. The difference between one laser and another has to do with the color of the light it emits, the characteristic of the light pulse, and the amount of energy it puts out. These three factors determine which skin target absorbs the laser or light beam, the size of the target in the skin that it will alter, and how much change it will produce. Some lasers are geared toward zapping red birthmarks, erasing redness from the cheeks, or banishing broken blood vessels. Others treat unwanted pigmentation, such as brown birthmarks, sun-induced brown spots, and tattoos. Still others remove excess hair, wrinkles, scars, stretch marks, and cellulite. The list is almost endless. To complicate things further, more and more doctors are offering treatments, like intense pulsed light, Thermage radio-frequency skin tightening, and Gentle Waves light-emitting diodes, that change the skin's texture and appearance using light and energy that aren't technically lasers. Taken together, these devices are called laser, light, and energy sources.

Handle with Care

As laser and light treatments become more popular and affordable, some people are beginning to view these devices as harmless gadgets that can be safely operated by anyone. It's true that skilled and experienced practitioners make zapping away hair, freckles, and fine lines look like child's play. Nevertheless, when these devices are used by someone who doesn't know enough about your complexion—or about the machine that he or she is using—lasers can injure the skin, leading to dark spots, permanent light spots, or scarring. Therefore, if you're considering one of these treatments, stay away from spas and "laser centers" that aren't doctor-supervised. I personally believe that it's best to have your procedure performed by either a doctor or a highly skilled nurse under the direct supervision of a doctor. Whoever your practitioner is, he or she should have extensive experience with the device that is being used on you.

I explained all of this and more to Gail. I told her that we could use bleaching creams and prescription retinoids from now until doomsday and, if we were lucky, see her hundreds of brown spots fade only partially. Gail wanted her spots *gone*, and she didn't want to watch her life pass her by while the creams gradually did their work. Once she got over her initial fear of the word *laser*, she asked me more about the treatment I was proposing. I told her that when we zap a spot with a Q-switched laser, the spot lightens immediately, so that it looks almost like a snowflake. This initial whitening clears within seconds and is replaced by redness, which lasts for a few hours. The brown spots then begin to darken, but only rarely do they scab.

Most of my patients tolerate the Q-switched laser treatment very well. Each zap stings a bit, so when we're talking about hundreds of spots, the procedure can be slightly uncomfortable. Nevertheless, no anesthesia, not even an anesthetic cream, is required for this treatment. About a week after the face is treated, the darkened areas flake off, leaving normally colored skin. (Spots on the hands and arms take about two weeks to clear up, and spots on the legs take about three treatments to achieve the desired amount of clearing.) In most cases we can erase the spots by about 80 to 90 percent. In general, the far-ther away you get from the face, the more difficult the spots are to clear up. (Don't let that discourage you from treating those areas, however; I see many women who think that their hands look about a decade older than their faces.)

I treated Gail on the day of our first consultation. Although we had time to address only a few of her spots, she was so thrilled with the results that she convinced her husband, Henry, to give it a go. We man-aged to zap away all his spots in just one round. Meanwhile, Gail con-tinued to see me every four to eight weeks, for a total of eight treatments, until we'd gotten rid of 90 percent of her spots. I've since learned that men's brown spots lighten more efficiently than women's do, sometimes requiring only one or two treatments; I'm not sure why this is so. Men, however, rarely seek treatment without some firm coaxing from the women in their lives.

As I mentioned earlier, light-source and energy devices vary tremendously. Most, such as those that treat sun-induced brown spots, "broken" (dilated) facial blood vessels, and excess hair, cause little discomfort. Some of the more aggressive resurfacing techniques, how-ever, require anesthesia and pain medications for a day or two after the procedure. A handful of machines, called ablative lasers, work by removing the upper layers of the skin, which means that you can end up so red and crusty that you'll want to hide out for a week or more. In contrast, the much more commonly used nonablative devices incite just enough minor injury below the skin's surface to help regenerate and re-form collagen, allowing you to return to your regular activities immediately. Most of these treatments yield very predictable results, which means that an expert dermatologist should be able to tell you in advance just how well you will respond to the treatment.

Will a Laser Treatment Work for *Me*?

If you're going to spend hundreds of dollars for each laser or energy-source treatment in a series, you want to hear that you're going to emerge looking younger or at least better than you did before. In most instances we can give such assurance. Although we can never determine how happy a patient will be with the results of a treatment, we can predict to a reasonable degree of certainty just how well brown spots will lighten, how well blood vessels will shrivel up and disappear, and so on. The outcome of a treatment depends on the following variety of factors:

What you are having treated. The results of most laser and light treatments are highly predictable and yield consistently good results. Q-switched lasers and intense pulsed light are used for removing lentigines, or sun-induced brown sun spots. Intense pulsed light, the long-pulsed diode, the alexandrite laser, and the Nd:YAG laser are used for hair removal. The CO_2, erbium, and fractional lasers, as well as the Plasma PSR, are used for resurfacing. Thermage and other skin-tightening devices are perhaps slightly less predictable, but as the technology improves, we can achieve increasingly better and more predictable results.

Your skin's condition now. The benefits you'll see are partly dependent on just how damaged your skin is before you embark on a treatment. If you have hundreds of dark brown spots, even a single treatment that lightens your spots by 50 percent will make a very

Myth Lasers, light, and energy sources are always a great replacement for traditional cosmetic surgery.

Truth In many instances this is the case. Plenty of people who might have considered cosmetic surgery years ago have found laser treatments to be an easier, safer, less painful alternative. We can lift the brows and firm up the jawline and neck somewhat by using skin-tightening devices like Thermage. Furthermore, those who aren't ready to commit to blepharoplasty might find that Thermage tightens the eye skin just enough to stave off surgery for some time. Others will find that a few quick passes with a laser to clear away fine lines and brown spots is all they really need. However, although these treatments are great for cleaning up the surface of the skin and firming up the collagen right below it, they're not a substitute for a surgical face-lift or eyelid lift, which can dramatically change the underlying structure of the face.

noticeable improvement. If, on the other hand, you begin with only twenty or so very light brown spots, that same 50 percent level of improvement will seem far less noticeable because you started out looking pretty good. You can apply the same logic to many of these treatments: you will see the greatest degree of improvement if you start with really damaged skin. As the saying goes, the closer you get to perfection, the harder it is to get there.

Your doctor's experience level. The doctor you choose should be very familiar with the device and should be able to tell you what you can expect from the treatment, how many sessions you will require, how far apart they should be, and what the healing process will be like. Your doctor should also be able to show you pictures of patients before and after and be willing to refer you to several patients whom he or she has treated with the device you are considering. If you wish, you should be able to chat with these patients and even meet one or two so that you can assess your dermatologist's work for yourself.

Anyone who has been paying attention to this issue in the last decade knows that lasers and energy-source devices are excellent tools for evening out brown splotches; resurfacing wrinkled, mottled skin; clearing broken facial blood vessels and facial redness; banishing unwanted hair; and even combating acne that lingers past adolescence. I've summarized the best treatments later (see "The Light Fantastic," page 211), but first I want to explore them in depth.

Brown Spots

What if you're plagued by increasing numbers of brown spots—just a few or many constellations of them—on your hands, legs, or arms? Even when unaccompanied by fine lines and wrinkles, lentigines can make you look far older than you actually are. Prescription retinoids work, but lightening takes six months to two years. Your spots also might be too stubborn or too numerous to budge with bleaching creams.

As my story of Gail and her husband attests, laser and light treatments can lighten or erase 80 to 90 percent of these spots in about three treatments, knocking years off your SVA. We have two different approaches to treating these spots: short-pulsed lasers, such as the ruby, alexandrite, and Nd:YAG lasers, treat one spot at a time. Because they work quickly, however, we can zap hundreds of spots—even an entire face and both hands—in a single treatment session. Patients tell me that the pain is minimal; they liken it to a finger being snapped against the skin. The discomfort lasts a few minutes to a maximum of one hour.

Our alternate tools are intense pulsed-light devices. These treat a bigger spot size and can be used to zap a bunch of individual spots or an entire large region—such as the face, the arms, or the chest—at one time. The area around each spot reddens for a few hours; meanwhile, your brown spots are temporarily covered with an ash color that lasts seconds to minutes after the treatment. After that, the spots increasingly darken, peaking by the end of the day. Facial spots actually remain a darker brown for about a week after each treatment (expect two weeks on the chest, the arms, and the hands and three weeks on the legs). Then the spots slowly flake off, leaving evenly colored skin. Patients tolerate all of the above treatments incredibly well and generally see no scabbing throughout the recovery period.

Red Blood Vessels

Another phenomenon that seems to get worse with age is the visible red blood vessels that crop up around the nose and the cheeks. They're very common, especially among people with fair complexions and those of Anglo-Saxon ancestry, which predisposes you to the problem. Since the symptoms are often associated with rosacea, these patients might have already tried prescription drugs like tetracycline, antibiotic pills such as minocycline or doxycycline, or prescription topicals such as MetroGel or Finacea. When these patients finally ask me whether there's anything else they can use, I always wish they had come to me sooner. That's because the prescription creams and pills for rosacea almost never help the redness, flushing, and broken blood vessels associated with the condition; they help only the pimples. Although anti-redness cleansers and lotions calm the skin a bit, it's usually not nearly enough for these cases.

The lasers we use to treat facial redness and blood vessels were first developed twenty years ago. Since then, they have been honed and perfected so that they now involve little or no downtime; require only three or four treatments; reduce redness, flushing, and broken vessels by as much as 90 percent; and routinely make patients far more attractive and happy. In short, they literally change people's lives. Pamela, an elementary school teacher who walked into my office wearing a flowing, old-fashioned skirt, a low bun in her hair, and a face as red as a fire engine, exemplifies this perfectly. A typical sturdy New Englander, fifty-two-year-old Pamela had naturally rosy cheeks—the kind strangers loved to pinch when she was a child.

During the past decade or so, the redness worsened, and her face would erupt into a flush at the slightest provocation. Now strangers would routinely ask her if she had a sunburn. She told me, "I just say the word *red* and my cheeks get red." You can imagine what happened when she stood in front of the world's most critical audience—a classroom of third graders—and attempted to impose any sort of order. "Teaching is hard enough," she said, "when your emotions aren't written all over your face. My cheeks feel hot; they even sting. This is ruining my life."

Considering how long Pamela had lived with this problem, it was amazing how quickly and dramatically we were able to improve the situation. We treated her three times with a pulsed dye laser. Pamela, who was never one to decline an educational opportunity, even turned her very first treatment into a field trip and invited her eight- and nine-year-old students to the laser clinic and the hospital to observe. The *Boston Herald*, a local daily newspaper, made the event into a front-page story. This thrilled me because we were able to convey a few important facts to the public: (1) Treating facial redness and broken blood vessels is a simple process that requires only a few visits. (2) It's barely painful; otherwise, Pamela wouldn't have been able to endure it in front of her students. (3) The procedure is a lot more affordable than most people think. (4) It really can be life altering. Pamela is living proof.

The pulsed dye laser, the first laser developed specifically for a medical use about twenty years ago, is still the treatment of choice for port-wine stain birthmarks. The latest enhanced version is also one of our favorite treatments for facial blood vessels, redness, and flushing. Also highly effective are the KTP laser and intense pulsed-light devices. Most of my patients find that a series of about three treatments yields dramatic results. Afterward, the area is red and a bit swollen for several hours—occasionally for a day or two—but generally you can go back to work the very next day.

Visible vessels and redness dissipate slowly but surely with each successive treatment. Once you achieve the degree of improvement you want, the vessels that have been cleared up stay away. However, because the treatment doesn't cure the condition that brought on the visible vessels, the vessels can reappear, along with redness, in the next one to three years. As a result, some patients opt for follow-up treatments once a year to keep things looking great. Others wait about three years to seek another series of treatments, until they see enough recurrent vessels or redness.

Excess Hair

Unwanted hair can be embarrassing and annoying to women of any age. If you're tired of shaving, waxing, or doing electrolysis, the latest lasers and light sources can feel like a godsend. Women with fair skin and dark hair have traditionally responded best. That's because most devices seek out the pigment in hair, causing heat damage to the hair shaft and follicle (without damaging the skin around it), so that the hair is either permanently gone or replaced by a much finer strand. In my office, we treat these patients with a long-pulsed diode, an alexandrite or a ruby laser, or an intense pulsed light device. New developments allow us to treat those with even the darkest skin or those who tan easily, typically with one of the long-pulsed Nd:YAG lasers, which achieve excellent results without the risk of laser-induced brown discoloration or the loss of pigment that the previously listed devices might cause. For most people, the treatments are mildly uncomfortable—comparable to being snapped by a rubber band—but rarely require anesthesia. (However, we always offer a topical anesthetic when treating large or sensitive areas.)

Although most people are thrilled with the results of laser hair removal, few ever find that their fuzz is totally gone. Your outcome will depend on your hair color and thickness, skin color, and treatment area. Nearly all of my patients initially find that they notice a temporary hair reduction. Even after the first treatment, their hair stays away for about six weeks before it regrows. The more treatments you have, the more lasting your hair reduction will be. To make sure that we catch the maximum number of hairs during their peak growing phase, we generally recommend having around six treatments four to six weeks apart. (Arm and leg hair is easiest to remove; underarm and bikini-line hair is next easiest; the hardest to remove is facial hair, especially hair above the upper lip and on the chin.) After completing a series of treatments, nearly 80 percent of those treated see a significant permanent reduction of unwanted hair. Finally, keep in mind that blond, white, and gray hair is much more difficult to remove. Our experience with these colors has been poor, so in these cases we recommend waxing, depilatories, tweezing, or electrolysis rather than laser or light-based treatment.

Myth   Lasers are great for permanently removing all unwanted hair.

Truth   This is a common misconception. Not long ago, a patient named Debbie told me how excited she was to start laser hair removal. "I want it all gone for good," she said. I hated to be the one to tell her that the absolute and total removal of hair is rare. The goal of these treatments is permanent hair-growth *reduction*. After treatment your hair will be lighter, finer, and much sparser, but most likely it won't be gone entirely. Expect approximately a 20 percent reduction with each treatment. That's what Debbie experienced, and she was still very pleased with the results. If you desire total, or almost total, hair removal, consider opting for more than the standard six treatments that we routinely recommend.

Sagging Skin

Brown spots, red blood vessels, and unwanted fuzz rank among the easiest issues to treat, but the sagging skin that gets worse with age has confounded doctors and patients alike for years. We used to always send people to plastic surgeons to lift and tighten jiggling jowls and tummies. Now, however, thanks to lasers and other energy-source devices, it's possible to improve these regions without the scalpel, stitches, or significant pain—and with little if any downtime.

One of the best known treatments, Thermage, has come a long way since it was first developed several years ago. Initially, its deep-heating radio frequency remodeled and regenerated collagen somewhat unpredictably and very painfully. A minority of patients saw satisfactory tightening, but most saw very little change at all. In the last few years the Thermage company has honed the technology significantly. Not only do the latest models work much better, the techniques for using them have also improved so much that these procedures are much more effective and comfortable. Our office headed a large international study that found that 90 percent of the fifty-seven hundred patients who used Thermage achieved the desired skin-tightening benefit. The procedure works beautifully for the cheeks, the jowl, the jawline, the upper neck, and the eyebrows, offering a nonsurgical alternative to the brow lift.

Like so many people, my patient Sondra, a tall, slim blonde who had just turned fifty-two, was skeptical that she would see much if any improvement without undergoing a face-lift. At the same time, she hated the idea of undergoing any type of surgical procedure. Nevertheless, she could no longer deny that every time she looked in the mirror, she saw her mother's face, complete with a developing jowl (sagging beneath her jaw and under her chin). Several years ago, Sondra had tried an early version of Thermage, with a small tip that treated the skin slowly, painfully, and unpredictably. It was not surprising that she hadn't been pleased with the results.

Meanwhile, her husband, a debonair, strikingly handsome businessman who looked years younger than his age, had been thrilled with the Thermage treatment I gave him a mere two years after Sondra's. By then, the device had been upgraded substantially so that the tip was larger and the treatment was more efficient and far less painful. As he was preparing for a follow-up treatment this past fall, he gave his wife a nudge. "You know," he said, "this could be just what you're looking for: a firmer jawline without a single incision and no recovery time." It took some convincing on his part, but she finally agreed, reluctantly, to give the treatment a try. Sondra was so pleased that she returned a year later for another round.

Thermage and its competitors just keep getting better. These days we have an ever-expanding range of specialized hand pieces in a variety of sizes that allow us to firm large nonfacial areas like the belly, the inner thighs, the upper inner arms, and even tiny, delicate areas such as droopy eyelids. There are also new competing tightening devices like Titan and ReFirme, which work similarly to Thermage, except that Titan heats with a broad-spectrum infrared lamp and ReFirme uses a combination of radio frequency and intense pulsed light. Keep in mind that these procedures can be painful (Titan and ReFirme less so than Thermage). Thermage requires only one treatment, whereas the others require two or three. You will see improvement the moment the procedure is finished, but the area will continue to tighten for six months afterward.

Resurfacing Lasers

All of the above devices are, for the most part, fairly gentle treatments that don't require you to hide out afterward. What about the ones that *do* come with significant downtime? Are they worth it? If you have decades worth of cumulative sun damage (brown spots or wrinkles) or prominent acne scarring, the more aggressive lasers might be just what you need.

Let's start with the mighty CO_2 laser, which resurfaces the entire face by removing the skin's wrinkled, scarred, and/or splotchy upper layers, ultimately revealing clear, baby-smooth skin underneath. Used by an expert, the ablative device produces dramatic improvement in

> **Myth** Why do I need lasers when I have all of these great skin creams?
>
> **Truth** It's a good question, considering that I've spent the first half of this book extolling the virtues of topical products. Of course, you don't *need* a laser treatment any more than you *need* Botox or cosmetic fillers. Nevertheless, laser treatments are infinitely more powerful than even the most effective cream, and they penetrate far below the skin's surface. If you don't want to wait for your topicals to work their magic, or if you want to see more dramatic change in your complexion, you might ask your dermatologist about lasers. This does not mean that you should give up your creams and lotions; they're excellent tools for maintaining the results of the laser treatments between appointments.

a single treatment. You can easily look ten to fifteen years younger in two weeks, which means that you don't have to return to the doctor for multiple treatments. Not for the faint of heart, this laser is best for those who have made up their minds to take the bull by the horns and make a significant positive change in the skin's destiny in one fell swoop. You must, I emphasize, seek a true pro, someone who has extensive experience with the CO_2 laser. Otherwise you could wind up permanently scarred. Even in the best cases, the treatment involves more than a week of recovery, during which time you'll be red, swollen, oozy, and crusted. With good wound care, however, you will heal beautifully and your skin will be smoother, brighter, and healthier looking that it has been in years.

What if you want some of the potency of a resurfacing laser but can afford to be laid up for only a few days afterward? With every passing year, we have many more options for resurfacing the skin without the risks and downtime of the CO_2 laser. The lasers and energy sources that are getting the most buzz right now include fractional treatments, like Fraxel, Fractional CO_2, and Active/Deep FX, as well as the Pearl laser and Portrait plasma energy technology. Fractional lasers injure only a fraction of the skin: tiny columns of the skin are lasered, leaving the surrounding areas intact for faster healing. You choose one of two protocols: The first involves six gentle treatments in about six months; each treatment results in three days of redness and swelling. The second entails one or two more aggressive treatments that leave the skin raw; it heals in about seven days.

Many of my patients also like the Portrait plasma technique, which pulses the skin with a high-energy nitrogen gas. Here, too, you have a choice of a series of gentle treatments with little downtime or one much more aggressive treatment. The latter leaves a paper-thin crust that acts as a protective dressing during the healing phase. Once the dressing falls off (after a week or so), you're left with a fresh, beautiful complexion.

The Sciton MicroLaserPeel, the Pearl laser, and the Active FX CO_2 laser offer patients a spectrum of choices. We program the instrument for the amount of improvement you want, and the laser does the rest. You can have one aggressive treatment with a week of downtime, or, like many of my patients, you may choose to do three gentle treatments in three months, which allows you to get back to work or resume your regular activities in three or four days.

All of these treatments are popular with women of all ages, because they essentially offer the ability to choose the strength of the resurfacing treatment.

Acne

Persistent acne is not a symptom that we normally associate with aging, but it can strike at any time—complete with the large pores and oily skin that we all thought would end after adolescence. The frustrating truth is that more and more women who have long since graduated from college suffer from unsightly pimples. Laser and light therapy for acne is still a developing field, but it's certainly worth a try if topical and oral medications don't help.

The most promising devices that are available right now are the mid-infrared lasers such as Smoothbeam, CoolTouch, and Aramis; photodynamic therapy; and a new device called Isolaz. The mid-infrared lasers seem to cause at least a temporary shrinkage of the sebaceous glands after a series of six sessions in six months. The procedure can be uncomfortable, and it usually leaves red spots that last for a few hours. However, I believe that they work best for inflammatory acne. Many of my patients also see improvement with intense pulsed light, pulsed dye lasers, blue light, or a combination of all three; their wavelengths kill acne-causing bacteria.

I and many other dermatologists are attempting to amplify the effects of these machines by first painting the skin with a topical solution that enhances the effect of light; we leave it on for an hour, then shine a laser or a light source on it. This is called photodynamic therapy (PDT). It kills bacteria and shrinks the oil glands in one shot, usually in three or more treatments performed every one to four weeks, followed by occasional maintenance treatments. Most of my patients tolerate PDT very well—although they might experience slight redness afterward—and see a significant reduction of their inflammatory acne. It's crucial that you continue to use your traditional acne treatments even while undergoing these light-based procedures, because even though they've yielded some success stories, the results with PDT and other laser and light treatments are quite uneven. These treatments are often not covered by insurance.

Lasers and Eye Safety

My patients often laugh when I hand them a pair of goggles just before beginning a laser procedure. It's a good way to diffuse the fear and tension that surrounds these treatments, but of course the funny-looking glasses serve a more important purpose: they protect the eyes—specifically the retina and the cornea—which can be permanently damaged from laser beams. Dermatologists take every precaution not to direct any light toward the eyes, but even an inadvertently reflected beam can be dangerous. Some laser injuries cause a burning sensation, but many can be painless, which means that you and your doctor might not realize that any injury has occurred until you see a black spot in the center of your vision. By then, it's usually too late to do anything to reverse the damage. The right protective eyewear—goggles, glasses, or metal shields that resemble gray suntan goggles—will defend you from possible damage. Safety is no laughing matter.

A new device is the Isolaz PPX system, a painless treatment that uses gentle suction to open the pores and clean out sebum and clogs. It's very effective for blackheads, whiteheads, red or pus-filled pimples, and, occasionally, cystic acne. Isolaz PPX also exposes the skin to intense pulsed light, which reduces skin inflammation, kills pimple-causing bacteria, and can shrink the oil glands. The suction offers a clean, hands-off approach to opening clogged pores, blackheads, and whiteheads. It's also safe for acne flare-ups during pregnancy. We usually recommend four or five treatments to be done either once a week or, more conveniently, every two or three weeks.

In our office, Isolaz treatments are done by medical aestheticians, who start by steaming the skin to open any blackheads or whiteheads. They then treat the entire face with three passes, using a smaller tip for the last pass to target problem areas. We finish the treatment with another steam. Though not effective for everyone, Isolaz has been quite successful in treating a variety of acne types, including blackheads and whiteheads, red inflamed pimples, and sometimes even deep acne nodules.

The Light Fantastic: Which Laser Treatment Is Right for You?

As promising as the laser and energy-source landscape is right now, it still can be devilishly hard to make sense of it. I know that all the information above might feel a bit overwhelming, so here's a summary of the most common skin issues for which our patients seek treatment and the lasers we tend to use for each. If you're even considering undergoing laser treatment, this will give you the information you need to have an educated conversation with your doctor.

Your diagnosis. You have constellations of brown spots (lentigines) on your face, hands, legs, and/or arms. Even when unaccompanied by fine lines and wrinkles, these can make you look far older than you actually are. Prescription retinoids work, but lightening takes six months to two years, and your spots might be too stubborn or too numerous to budge with bleaching creams.

Consider. Short-pulsed lasers, such as the ruby, alexandrite, and Nd:YAG lasers, treat one spot at a time. Because they work quickly, however, we can zap hundreds of spots, even an entire face and both hands, in a single treatment session. We also use intense pulsed light devices, which treat a bigger spot size and can be used to fade a bunch of individual spots or an entire large region—such as the face, the arms, or the chest—at one time.

Your diagnosis. Perhaps you've been noticing clusters of tiny red blood vessels forming around your nose and on your cheeks, or maybe you're troubled by increasing facial redness or flushing, whether from rosacea or not. Although topical anti-redness formulas can help to subdue the color slightly, the only way to take care of the problem is through laser and light-source treatments.

Consider. The pulsed dye laser, the first laser that was developed specifically for medical use, is still the treatment of choice for port-wine stain birthmarks. The latest enhanced version is also one of our favorite treatments for visible facial blood vessels, redness, and flushing. Also highly effective are the KTP laser and intense pulsed-light devices. Most of my patients find that a series of about three treatments yields dramatic results.

Your diagnosis. Parts of your face and body, especially your jawline, neck, forehead, eyelids, belly, upper inner arms, and thighs, have begun to droop and crinkle with age. Even if you're on a good topical daily regimen and have begun to use fillers, you're troubled by the drawn, early sagging that you see when you look in the mirror.

Consider. Skin-tightening treatments like Thermage, Titan, or ReFirme are the best. Thermage uses deep-heating radio frequency and infrared light to remold and tighten the collagen below the skin's surface and stimulate new collagen growth over time in areas as small as around the eyes and as large as the belly. You will see improvement the moment the procedure is finished, but the area will continue to tighten for six months afterward.

Treating Scars with the Pulsed Dye Laser

ike unwanted hair and acne, scars aren't symptoms that we automatically associate with aging. However, most people do tend to accumulate them as the years go by, due to surgical procedures and unexpected traumas. We've had tremendous success treating scars with the pulsed dye laser. A series of treatments not only flattens and fades red, raised scars but also helps to decrease their discomfort. This makes the pulsed dye laser an excellent tool for those who have had face-lifts, breast reduction surgery, or thyroid and neck procedures or for those who have been in car accidents that resulted in lacerations. The treatments do cause bruises that last for four to seven days, but the ultimate rewards are life changing.

Your diagnosis. Unwanted hair on your face, legs, arms, underarms, or bikini line can be a nuisance at any age. If you're tired of shaving, waxing, or doing electrolysis, laser and light hair removal can offer a better, long-term solution.

Consider. A long-pulsed diode, an alexandrite laser, or a ruby laser work well, or try an intense pulsed light device if you have dark hair and fair skin. If you have darker skin or tan easily, we recommend one of the long-pulsed Nd:YAG lasers, which achieve excellent results without the risk of laser-induced brown discoloration or loss of pigment, which the previously listed devices might cause. Unfortunately, blond, white, and gray hair is much more difficult to remove. Our experience with these colors has been poor, so in these cases we recommend waxing, depilatories, tweezing, or electrolysis.

Your diagnosis. You have persistent acne that is often accompanied by large pores and oily skin. Many patients erroneously assume that pimples fade away after adolescence. In fact, more and more women who have long since graduated from college suffer from unsightly pimples. Laser and light therapy for acne is still a developing field, but it's certainly worth a try if topical and oral medications don't help.

Consider. Infrared laser treatments like Smoothbeam, CoolTouch, and Aramis; photodynamic therapy; and Isolaz work best. Another alternative (which you can use alone or in combination with the lasers above) is light therapy: blue light, pulsed dye lasers, or intense pulsed light. Their wavelengths kill acne-causing bacteria. Although light-based acne procedures have yielded some success stories, the results are quite uneven, and the treatments are often not covered by insurance. New on the horizon is Isolaz PPX, a painless treatment that uses gentle suction plus intense pulsed light to clean out sebum and clogs, kill bacteria, and possibly shrink the oil glands. This makes it very effective for blackheads, whiteheads, red or pus-filled pimples, and, occasionally, cystic acne. It's not effective for everyone, but we have been quite pleased with the results of Isolaz treatments.

Your diagnosis. You have decades worth of cumulative sun damage, including many brown spots and some wrinkles, or perhaps you have poor skin texture and acne scarring. Either way, you'd rather have one treatment and then hide out for a couple of weeks than opt for gentler treatments that could take weeks or months to make any significant difference.

Consider. The mighty CO_2 laser resurfaces the entire face by removing the skin's wrinkled, scarred, and/or splotchy upper layers, ultimately revealing clear, baby-smooth skin underneath. Used by an expert, the ablative device produces dramatic improvement in a single treatment. You can easily look ten to fifteen years younger in two weeks, which means that you don't have to return to the doctor for multiple treatments. Seek out a true expert who has extensive experience with the CO_2 laser. Otherwise you could end up permanently scarred. Even in the best cases, the treatment involves more than a week of recovery, during which time you'll be red, swollen, oozy, and crusted. With good wound care, however, you will heal beautifully and your skin will be smoother, brighter, and healthier looking than it has been in years.

Your diagnosis. You don't like your skin texture. Perhaps you have decades worth of cumulative sun damage, including many brown spots and some wrinkles. Maybe you have acne scarring, less extensive freckling, or fine lines. Although topical creams could help, you'd prefer not to wait for them to work. On the other hand, you're too squeamish, or simply too busy, to undergo any treatment that will leave you laid up for more than a few days.

Consider. You should use one of the devices that work a little less dramatically than the CO_2 laser. These include fractional treatments like the Fraxel, the Fractional CO_2, and the Active FX lasers as well as the Pearl laser and the Portrait plasma energy treatment. Fractional lasers injure only a fraction of the skin, which allows for faster healing. The Portrait plasma technique pulses the skin with a high-energy nitrogen gas, leaving a paper-thin crust that acts as a protective dressing during the healing phase. Once the dressing falls off (after a week or so), you're left with a fresh, beautiful complexion. There is also the Sciton MicroLaserPeel. You can have one aggressive treatment with a week of downtime, or you may choose to do three gentle treatments in three months, which allows you to get back to work or resume your regular activities in three or four days. The Pearl laser works similarly.

Doctor's Orders

All lasers, no matter how effective, come with an important caveat: even if your dermatologist manages to smooth away decades' worth of sun damage, you will continue to age after treatment. New lines, broken blood vessels, and brown spots will return eventually, so most patients opt for follow-up visits from one year to several years after their first round of treatments. Here's the good news: you can keep the signs of aging from coming back too quickly by practicing good sun protection 365 days per year. That means avoiding exposure when the sun is strongest and highest in the sky and slathering on sunscreen every time you do venture outside. Keep in mind that freshly lasered skin is especially vulnerable to harsh ultraviolet rays, so depending on which treatment you have, you'll need to be even more careful about covering up during the week or two afterward.

The Vein Game

Dermatologists can do incredible things to the surface of the skin using lasers and other energy devices, but what about what lies beneath? Two of the most common gripes I hear from my patients involve veins and cellulite, both of which plague women disproportionately more than men. Unfortunately, both also only worsen with age. I want to start by talking about veins, since we dermatologists have several effective weapons in our arsenal to take care of them. (Cellulite, unfortunately, is a little more stubborn; we'll get to that later.)

Myth My skin is so damaged that there is no point even starting with lasers.

Truth I hear this frequently from my patients, particularly those with more mature skin and decades of accumulated sun damage. We doctors have many, many different lasers and light sources at our disposal these days. Some are extremely gentle and, it is true, might make little difference in extremely damaged skin, but others are powerful enough to take care of the most advanced wrinkles, sagging, and brown spots. Even if your regimen of topical creams has stopped working wonders, the right laser can make a world of difference.

Let me tell another story about a longtime patient of mine. Until recently, Denise had come to see me about fairly standard issues. She was diligent about scheduling skin cancer screenings, she routinely asked me to recommend cleansers and treatment lotions, and she had just begun to use a prescription retinoid that I recommended for her emerging fine lines. Denise was not especially interested in going beyond the topical realm of skin care—until she went swimsuit shopping a few weeks before going on a vacation to the Caribbean. She had been aware of the spider veins webbing her thighs for years, but somehow she didn't recall their being quite *this* visible until she stood under those notoriously unflattering fluorescent lights. "Dr. Dover," she said when she stopped by a day later, "I'm a little desperate. Is there anything I can use on these veins to make them go away?"

If you happen to have extremely pale skin like Denise, rubbing on a coat of self-tanner might make your veins a little less starkly obvious. Other than that, however, there's no topical formula that can help. Denise was quite pleased to learn that regardless of whether veins are thick and ropy, tiny and red (the facial kind), or purple and spidery, it's never been easier to treat them, right in the doctor's office. Lasers and other light sources offer a quick, lasting fix for facial red blood vessels and flushing. Although these painless veins might start mildly enough, they often worsen with age, becoming especially visible along the sides of the nose and on the cheeks. As anyone who suffers from them knows, alcohol consumption, smoking, and sun and heat exposure only worsen the problem. The best treatment is intense pulsed light and the KTP or pulsed dye laser. For the bluish veins that occasionally appear around the eyes, at the temples, and on the forehead I prefer the long-pulsed Nd:YAG laser. After an average of three treatments, we can banish the problem completely, with only a day or so of minor downtime.

Although lasers and light sources are highly effective for treating broken facial blood vessels, sclerotherapy is the gold standard for 98 percent of leg veins, whether the extremely fine kind or the big varicose veins. Starting with the largest veins and working our way down to the smallest, we inject a variety of different sclerosing agents, such as saline, glycerin, or Sotradecol. This safely irritates the vein wall, causing the vessel to collapse and also causing inflammation. The vessel, in turn, shrivels up and becomes reabsorbed by the body within a few weeks to a few months. Depending on how many veins you have, the procedure can be done in a thirty-minute treatment session, but it is usually done in a series of treatments. The injections sting a bit, but most patients tolerate it very well. After treatment we always wrap the legs in ace bandages or pressure stockings for at least several days. This keeps the vessels collapsed and helps to prevent them from reopening. Following, I've listed the most common types of visible veins, what each looks like, and how to make them all go away.

Spider Leg Veins

What they are. Much like facial veins, spider leg veins are red and tiny, about the width of a strand of hair.

How to treat them. For ultrafine spider veins, which are too small to fit a needle into, we generally use lasers and light sources. Two or three treatments are necessary. It is absolutely essential—even more than when you're undergoing facial laser treatments—not to be tan when you are using a laser on spider leg veins, because the risk of brown discoloration is very high. When it does occur, it can take months to clear. For small spider veins that are big enough to pierce with a tiny sclerotherapy needle, sclerotherapy injections are the treatment of choice.

Blue Reticular Leg Veins

What they are. Flat and painless, blue reticular leg veins emerge in a netlike pattern, most often in women with fair skin. They're typically more visible when the body is cold.

How to treat them. Sclerotherapy is once again the therapy of choice. A series of treatments is required. When treating these slightly larger veins, I require my patients to wear special pressure wraps and leg hose for several days afterward.

Varicose Veins

What they are. Varicose veins are blue, squishable veins that, when engorged with blood, can be as thick as your baby finger. Although they're sometimes painless, they're often associated with leg aches, especially near the end of the day, after you've been standing for long periods. Those who are overweight, who have a history of deep vein thrombosis (leg clots), or whose family members have varicose veins are especially prone. (Patients often say to me, "I remember that my grandmother had things that felt like worms on the backs of her calves when I was a little girl.")

How to treat them. Compression sclerotherapy is one of the most popular and effective treatments for big, ropy veins. After a sclerother-

Myth Using sclerotherapy to treat my leg veins is old-fashioned and painful. Lasers are more cutting-edge and effective.

Truth Lasers offer an advanced, efficient way to treat many skin issues, like wrinkles, sagging, and unwanted hair. They can also be used for leg veins, but in this case, sclerotherapy remains the gold standard. By collapsing the vein wall with glycerin or other medical solutions, we can safely treat 98 percent of cases, usually in a series of sessions and with just a bit of stinging. I typically reserve lasers, which are less effective, for vessels that are too small for a needle.

apy injection, we wrap the legs in pressure stockings for three days to a week, but patients who suffer from chronic varicose veins should wear these stockings daily. (The stockings come in a variety of colors and styles, and they actually make the leg feel much more comfortable, even after a long day of standing.) These stockings are great at preventing leg swelling and aching even for those with normal leg veins. When I wear them, I feel like running a marathon at the end of the day.

A popular alternative treatment for varicose veins was, until very recently, leg-vein stripping. This surgical procedure requires incisions to be made in the skin at intervals along the length of the vein, and small portions of the vein are then extracted. It's usually done under anesthesia and leaves a scar at each incision.

Dermatologists are increasingly turning to much less invasive procedures for this condition, however. The first of these, ambulatory phlebectomy, still utilizes incisions to remove segments of the dilated vein, but the cuts are tiny, leaving almost invisible scars. The latest development, called endovenous phlebectomy, uses ultrasound to guide the physician, who uses either laser or radio-frequency probes to zap the walls of large veins, causing them to collapse. Before the procedure, the doctor anesthetizes the overlying skin, makes a single incision in the groin or at the very end of the vein, then inserts the probe down the leg vein, leaving only one very small scar. It has at least a 90 percent success rate, and patients can return to work and resume regular activities within a day or two.

Cellulite: The Dreaded Dimples

If veins are one of the most fixable issues that people complain about, cellulite represents one of the most elusive. My patient Susan can attest to that. At age forty-five, the part-time yoga instructor and compulsive jogger had the kind of body that all her friends and clients envied. This was hardly a surprise, considering that she ate mostly vegetables, fruits, and whole grains. When Susan visited me recently, I immediately spotted twenty different issues that we could address to make her look better, starting with her lingering acne, her imperfect facial texture, and her emerging brown spots. "I'm not worried about those things at all," she insisted. "*This* is what concerns me." Susan revealed a patch of dimpling fat that covered the back of her thigh, explaining that its appearance had only gotten worse after a round of liposuction several years before. Now she wanted my help.

I had a few suggestions for Susan, but I couldn't make any promises because, as Susan had seen firsthand, not even the most invasive treatments can do much for stubborn cellulite. This is a condition that is as common as it is tough to treat. Cellulite affects more than 90 percent of women over the age of eighteen. It's almost universally a female issue because of the way that women's fat is distributed and because women tend to have more body fat than men have. The subcutaneous layer of fat is compartmentalized in between vertical bands of fibrous tissue. As fat accumulates, especially in areas like the buttocks, the back of the thighs, and the belly, the fibrous bands around it begin to pucker and dimple, and voilà: cellulite.

It is no surprise that the cellulite cream business is a billion-dollar industry. Many of these formulas contain aminophylline, caffeine, retinol, and other so-called active ingredients, many of which, frankly, I've never heard of. I haven't seen any good data that show that even one of these creams works. Then there's mesotherapy, a procedure *not* approved by the FDA, which involves the injection of detergents that are designed to melt away fat. If these substances even work, how safe are they? What happens to the melted fat? Does it come back? Until someone produces properly done scientific studies that show that this procedure is safe and effective, I'll withhold judgment, and I will continue telling my patients to avoid it. (The Brazilian government recently banned mesotherapy. That's a pretty bad sign, since Brazil rarely bans anything!)

Because so many people are paying good money for treatments that turn out to be ineffective (or potentially dangerous), it's no wonder that the handful of therapies that hold even a little bit of promise are getting so much attention. I'm pleased to say that the latest round of cellulite-fighting lasers and energy sources do offer some hope. All FDA-approved, the VelaSmooth, TriActive, and Accent devices are somewhat successful in recontouring puckers of fat. VelaSmooth uses suction and radio frequency, TriActive uses a combination of suction and diode laser, and Accent uses radio frequency. (The suction component of these is essentially an updated version of Endermologie, which offers a high-tech rubdown that's designed to break up pockets of fat.)

There's more exciting news on the horizon: several companies, such as UltraShape and LipoSonics, are developing devices that use techniques like high-frequency ultrasound and shock waves, while others like Zeltiq use localized cooling to dissolve fat. These might help cellulite, but what's even more thrilling is that they actually reduce fat—and potentially your waistline. One of these companies has data showing that the technique removes an inch off your waistline in a single treatment. It's not quite liposuction, but it's much easier and has decent results. None of these is yet approved by the FDA. Still, the pace of discovery is rapid and the results are very promising.

9

Surgical Cosmetic Procedures

When cocktail party conversations turn to beauty treatments, few topics stir up as much passion and controversy as cosmetic surgery. Think about the tabloid magazines you read in line at the supermarket and the gossip shows on TV. If they're not talking about which celebrities are dating or divorcing, they're usually speculating about which actress looks suspiciously as if she's had a face-lift or which one appears to have sprouted fuller breasts, seemingly overnight.

When I have serious, in-depth conversations with my patients about their own feelings toward cosmetic surgical procedures, I find that some have strong sentiments for or against these treatments, but many others aren't quite sure where they stand. What about you? How do you feel about cosmetic surgery, and how informed are you? Now's your chance to find out; just take the quiz below.

1. The best way to determine how you'll look after a face-lift is to

   A. Examine a friend who has had the procedure done

    B. See an expert and have him or her show you how you might look after the procedure. The doctor will most likely have you hold a mirror and gently pull the edges of your face and neck until the skin looks smooth.

    C. Just go ahead and have the surgery done—it's a fairly minor procedure

2. Which of the following will a face-lift or an eye lift *not* accomplish?

    A. A redraping of the skin

    B. A dramatic improvement of skin texture and quality

    C. A reduction of wrinkles

3. Compared to a conventional brow lift, an endoscopic brow lift is

    A. A less invasive procedure

    B. A more invasive procedure

    C. A brow lift that is performed with lasers

4. Blepharoplasty surgery addresses the

    A. Abdomen

    B. Upper arms

    C. Eyes

5. Liposuction is a good option when you

    A. Don't have time to diet and exercise

    B. Need to lose a quick thirty pounds

    C. Can't lose one or two pockets of fat despite your healthy lifestyle and regular exercise program

6. Abdominoplasty (a tummy tuck) is

    A. A pretty invasive surgical procedure

    B. So minimally invasive that some women can return to work the next day

    C. No longer recommended—energy sources like Thermage offer the same results with far less downtime

7. What is the main downside to hair transplantation?

   A. Even when doctors use the latest techniques available, the results look fake.

   B. The surgery is costly and tedious.

   C. Both of the above

8. Which surgical procedure is more involved?

   A. Breast augmentation

   B. Breast reduction

   C. They're about comparable.

9. Given the option between a cutting-edge surgical procedure and one that's been around for years, which should you choose?

   A. The newest one

   B. The tried-and-true procedure

   C. Research both as much as possible, then make a decision

10. The benefit to choosing cosmetic surgery over less invasive procedures like lasers or injectables is that surgical results

    A. Will last longer

    B. Will last forever

    C. Are always better than those of less invasive procedures

Answers

1. B: Although you can look to a friend for reference, her appearance has little to do with how *you'll* look after a face-lift. Notwithstanding all of those plastic surgery reality shows, having a face-lift—or any other surgical procedure—is nothing to take lightly. To get an idea of how a face-lift might affect your face, you can start by gently pulling the edges of your face and neck back in front of a mirror. Then talk to a doctor you trust to learn more.

2. B: Done properly, these surgical procedures will indeed redrape the skin, smoothing wrinkles in the process. However, they'll do

nothing for the textural and pigmentary sun damage you've accumulated over the years. For that, look to treatment creams, lasers, chemical peels, and/or microdermabrasion.

3. A: During an endoscopic brow lift, your surgeon will make several very tiny incisions in the scalp, use a small viewing probe to pull the sagging areas, and snip the muscles that cause frown lines. This makes it a less invasive surgery than a traditional brow lift. Recovery time is far less, but keep in mind that this procedure's results (which do nothing for horizontal forehead lines) are less dramatic and shorter-lived.

4. C: One of the most commonly performed invasive procedures, blepharoplasty (or eyelid surgery) rejuvenates the eyes by removing excess eyelid skin and/or the bulges of fat appearing on either the eyelids or under the eyes. Occasionally it also tightens the muscles beneath the eyes.

5. C: Liposuction is not an alternative to working out or having a healthy diet, and it's not for people who have a large amount of weight to lose. Instead, I recommend it for patients who have a stubborn area of fat—belly fat or saddlebags, for example— that won't budge, no matter what they do.

6. A: Abdominoplasty is a major operation that removes excess skin and sometimes fat; it's definitely not a lunchtime procedure. The results are dramatic, much more than anything a skin-tightening procedure can offer.

7. B: Hair transplantation is expensive and time-consuming. For those who suffer from hair loss, however, the procedure can be worth it. Doctors now use natural-looking micrografts rather than obvious hair plugs. The results can be so exceptional that even I can't tell that it's been done.

8. B: Making the breasts smaller is far more involved than making them larger. Reduction surgery generally requires more extensive incisions and stitches. It also leaves more scars, which are visible, sometimes painful, and occasionally red and thickened,

and they often require treatment with steroid injections or lasers.

9. C: When it comes to cosmetic surgery, or any dermatological procedure, latest doesn't always mean greatest. You're better off doing your own research and gathering opinions from a few trusted doctors as well as from their patients.

10. A: In general, if you see a good doctor, cosmetic surgery will give you more dramatic, longer-lasting results than lasers or injectables do. The results won't last forever, however, so many patients prefer the more subtle alterations of Botox, fillers, and lasers to the sudden changes brought on by the scalpel.

Mindy's Story: When a Face-Lift Is the Right Treatment

Assuming that you've read the first eight chapters of this book (or even just skimmed them), you know that good skin care is the crux of my anti-aging plan. If you wash your face morning and night with a cleanser, apply the right cocktail of treatment products, guard against too much sunlight exposure, and use sunscreen, your complexion will reward you by looking smoother, brighter, tighter, and more vibrant

---

Myth The newer a procedure is, the better it must be.

Truth Doctors and patients alike are fortunate to have an ever-widening array of new treatments from which to choose. With all of the hoopla that accompanies each new topical product, laser, or surgical procedure, it's tempting to think that *new* always equals *best*. To that I say, buyer beware. No matter how modified or improved a particular treatment claims to be, it's had less time out in the world than the older, time-tested treatments. Is an endoscopic brow lift better than the conventional kind? Are the results as good, and do they last as long? Is SmartLipo necessarily any more effective than the traditional liposuction that we've been using for years? Maybe it is, maybe it isn't. Only time will tell.

than you ever imagined. If topicals alone aren't lowering your SVA, we have an array of techniques (injectable fillers, Botox, and lasers) that do an amazing, quick job of jump-starting the improvement.

That's what Mindy counted on when she visited my office last year. Bright, witty, and sixty-one years old, Mindy had stopped by to see a general dermatologist for a basic skin-cancer check. As she left his exam room, she spotted me in the corridor and couldn't believe it when I remembered her from the time I'd met her a decade earlier. I often forget patients' names, but I almost never forget a face—a good thing for a dermatologist whose livelihood depends on recognizing facial patterns.

Mindy and I stood in the corridor catching up for a minute, and she finally asked what I thought she should do to look younger. I asked her if she had thirty minutes free and offered to fit her in for a consultation between my appointments. She agreed and stepped into our private waiting room until I called her into my office a few minutes later.

I started the way I always do: handing her a mirror and asking her to show me what about her skin bothered her the most. She didn't hesitate, pointing to her deep nasolabial and melolabial folds and the pronounced sagging of her lower face and neck. Mindy had been wondering for years if she was a candidate for Botox, fillers, laser treatments, or even a face-lift. She could definitely have benefited from Botox or fillers, but she really didn't need laser treatments, because her skin tone and color were surprisingly even and smooth. Before we even considered injectables, however, I suggested that she see two of the best face-lift surgeons in Boston. (Mindy was a wise woman who always insisted on getting at least two opinions.) As we wrapped up, I recommended a daily skin-care regimen

Myth I've heard of doctors who say they can lift the breasts using Botox.

Truth So have I. In just the right scenario, Botox can alter the muscles of the chest to temporarily elevate the breasts. For the most part, however, these claims are a myth. For most patients, I'd have to use large, very costly amounts of Botox to achieve any sort of lift. Even then, the change would be barely noticeable.

to maintain the quality of her complexion. In the end, she decided to have a face-lift, and she was thrilled to see that her sagging decreased dramatically. Once she healed, she returned to me to talk about what else we could do to make her look even better. A few months later, she did, in fact, come in for a bit of Botox and filler to take care of her remaining creases and folds.

One of the reasons I tell this story is that it raises an increasingly perplexing question: What is cosmetic surgery, anyway? Until several years ago, the answer was very clear. Cosmetic surgery involved scalpels and anesthesia and weeks of postoperative recovery time, and for many people it was prohibitively expensive. However, the lines have blurred quite a bit since then. In just the past ten years or so, a growing class of treatments has emerged that straddle the line between the surgical and the nonsurgical. For the most part, Botox, injectable fillers, lasers, light, and radio-frequency treatments are relatively noninvasive, speedy, affordable procedures that require little or no recovery time. They involve no

Least invasive
Cleanser
Sunscreen
Prescription and over-the-counter topical treatments
Microdermabrasion Vibraderm
Superficial acid peels
Botox
Fillers
Sclerotherapy
Lasers and light sources to treat facial brown and red discoloration, facial vessels, and remove hair
Nonsurgical skin tightening
Laser skin rejuvenation
Liposuction
Eyelid lift
Hair transplantation
Classic face-lift and other traditional cosmetic surgeries, like brow lift, tummy tuck, and so on
Most invasive

The spectrum of dermatologic treatment, from cleansers to cosmetic surgery.

scalpels and only occasionally require anesthesia. Yet depending on whom you ask, a few of these treatments—especially some fillers and the more aggressive laser procedures like CO_2 resurfacing—do fall under the term *cosmetic surgery.* The semantics don't matter nearly as much as this truth: most of these new procedures are quick, performed in-office, and yield spectacular results that can change your appearance and your life with little drama or trauma.

It's little wonder, then, that these minimally invasive treatments are increasing in popularity year after year. In fact, if you look at the spectrum of currently available anti-aging options shown in the chart on page 229, you'll find many, many more on the less invasive side than on the more invasive side. The chart illustrates what I mean.

As Mindy's story proves, the treatments on the top portion of the spectrum don't (pardon the pun) cut it for everyone. Sometimes, *true* cosmetic surgery—the kind that does involve scalpels and anesthesia and postoperative wound care—really is your best approach. Injectables and lasers, for example, can't enlarge or reduce the size of your breasts, change the shape of your nose, or remove large portions of skin or fat (at least not yet). Although you can alleviate some sagging with tightening devices like Thermage, more significant sagging of the face and the neck usually requires a face-lift. Expertly injected Botox and skin-tightening procedures can lift the eyebrows a few millimeters, but anything more extensive usually necessitates a brow lift. That's why we have an eye plastic surgeon at our center and why I work very closely with the best plastic surgeons in Boston. We don't hesitate to refer our patients to these doctors when they require the kind of invasive surgical procedures, like eyelid lifts or face-lifts, that our arsenal of less invasive tools just can't accomplish.

Thanks, in part, to certain reality TV shows that depict ordinary, everyday people undergoing face-lifts, nose jobs, and tummy tucks (sometimes, horrifyingly, in one tidy half-hour episode!), down-to-earth women who thought they'd never consider anything more invasive than microdermabrasion are suddenly asking me about cosmetic surgery. Don't get me wrong, these procedures are nothing to take lightly—my colleagues and I bristle when we watch the doctors on these TV shows talk about surgery as if they're hairstylists who are discussing the proper placement of highlights. But let's face it: for better or for worse, appearance counts more than ever these days, and the beauty-standard bar keeps being raised higher and higher. There are times when going under the knife is absolutely warranted. Therefore, although I've devoted the bulk of this book to skin care and the scores of simple *non*surgical approaches to anti-aging—the kind that require little more time than it takes to eat lunch—I'd be doing you a disservice if I didn't include a chapter on the most popular cosmetic surgical procedures, should you choose to go down that road.

Face-Lift

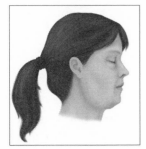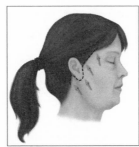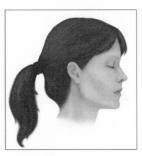

Before surgery   Incision and direction of facial lift   After surgery

Before and after drawings of a face-lift.

What it is. A face-lift is a surgical procedure that redrapes the skin of the lower part of the face and neck, making it tighter and smoother. (Less common is the so-called mid-face-lift, which firms sagging skin in the central portion of the face.) To get an idea of how you would look after a face-lift, stand in front of a mirror and gently pull the edges of your face and neck back and up until your loose skin looks smooth and taut.

    What to expect. Typically, your surgeon will put you to sleep—or at least into a twilight state—with either a general anesthesia or a combination of a local anesthesia and a sedative. Your surgeon will carefully examine your face to determine just how dramatically your skin should be pulled back to make it look smooth, not pleated. Depending on what areas require lifting, an incision will be made that runs from the temples to just in front of your ears, then around and behind the ears into the hairline. Excess skin will be removed, then the remaining skin will be pulled back and upward and then stitched along the incision line.

Pros. Performed by a true master, a face-lift can dramatically eliminate the most stubborn areas of sagging skin in one fell swoop, smoothing wrinkles and creases in the process. Although the operation doesn't stop the clock, it does knock years off your face. Thus, when you start to sag again, you'll do so from a new, younger baseline.

Cons. The dramatic change brought on by a face-lift might be a serious drawback for women who prefer subtler, more incremental change. If the procedure is performed by a surgeon who is inexperienced, overly aggressive, or not particularly artistic or skilled, you could wind up with a severe, overly pulled-back face, with visible scars, or worse. Many patients are not wild about the idea of being

---

Mini-Lift

For anyone who is looking for a more dramatic treatment than lasers or cosmetic injectables, but who shudders at the idea of having a full-fledged face-lift, the term *mini-lift* can sound like a rather appealing middle ground. The procedure entails making smaller incisions, pulling the skin less dramatically, and typically comes with a shorter postoperative recovery period. Yet even though the so-called mini-lift, sometimes known as the S-Lift, sounds promising, weigh your options before you commit.

My close friend and colleague Jay Burns, a plastic surgeon in Dallas, Texas, argues that the mini-lift "yields mini results—and maximum disappointment." Based on the experiences of my own patients, I'd say he's right. To use a familiar analogy, let's say you want to paint your house. One painter comes along and says that he's going to carefully sand the exterior, apply a layer of primer, then put on a coat of paint. Another painter says, "Forget about sanding and priming—I'll just put on one really nice coat of paint, charge you half, and *trust me,* your house will look as good as new." If you're going to go to the trouble of rehabilitating your house—or, even more important, your face—why not do it right so that you can enjoy lasting results for years to come? Why endure the sedation, cutting, bruising, and downtime associated with surgery, for mini results? There are doctors who say that this procedure is a good choice for those with only a bit of sagging. In my opinion, these people would be better off starting with a no-downtime treatment like Thermage, Titan, or ReFirme.

sedated or enduring two or more weeks of bruising, swelling, and the general recovery that follows the surgery. (If you aren't in the best health, you might not be a suitable candidate for such a big procedure.) Keep in mind that even though a face-lift tightens sun-damaged sagging skin, it does absolutely nothing to improve the overall health of the skin. Essentially, if you have sagging, sun-damaged skin when you undergo the procedure, you'll have tight, sun-damaged skin when the healing process is over. That's why everyone who has a face-lift should also embark on a great skin-care program and consider booking the appropriate in-office treatments to improve the complexion's color, tone, and texture.

Who benefits most. A face-lift is best for those who have significant sagging of the middle and lower parts of the face and neck. In cases of profound sagging, we can do nonsurgical skin-tightening procedures such as Thermage instead, but you just won't get the same level of results as you will from a well-done face-lift.

Brow Lift

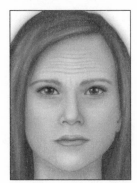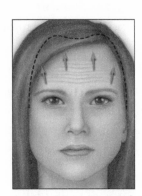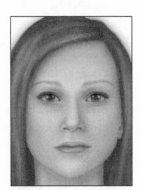

Before   Incision site and direction of   After
                  forehead lift

Before and after drawings of a brow lift.

What it is. A brow lift is a surgical procedure that helps to rejuvenate the upper face by doing as the name says: elevating drooping eyebrows while smoothing the deep lines and furrows in the forehead. (It's also called a forehead lift.) Some patients opt to have a brow lift along with a face-lift and/or a blepharoplasty (eyelid surgery).

What to expect. This is a big procedure and not for the faint of heart. Generally, your doctor will make an incision from ear to ear across the front of the scalp, which is hidden just behind the hairline. Through this incision, your surgeon can alter the muscles that cause horizontal forehead wrinkles and scowling. A strip of excess skin is excised, and then your forehead skin is pulled back and sutured down into place. Postoperative recovery—during which time you'll experience bruising, swelling, and possibly numbness and tingling—lasts about six weeks. You'll probably look respectable enough to go out about two weeks after the procedure.

Pros. A brow lift eliminates sagging skin and forehead wrinkles, and, perhaps most important, it elevates the eyebrows quite dramatically. The procedure is perfect for those who are looking for significant eyebrow elevation, more than can be achieved with a nonsurgical skin-tightening treatment like Thermage, Titan, or ReFirme.

Cons. The incisions are large, and the postoperative recovery (which includes discomfort, swelling, and bruising) is significant and certainly not pleasant. People who have high foreheads or thin hair that they usually wear back might not like the fact that the operation raises the hairline. Furthermore, after the procedure is over, the hair around the incision might temporarily thin or fall out. The area around the scar and on the top of the head is often numb for months—and occasionally forever. Perhaps most alarming is that a brow lift done too aggressively can leave you with a permanently surprised look.

Who benefits most. An expert dermatologist can raise your eyebrows modestly and eliminate even the deepest lines with Botox. Tightening devices like Thermage and ReFirme can modestly remedy sagging skin on the forehead as well. However, if you don't like the idea of returning for regular follow-up visits, or if your sagging is too far gone for those minimally invasive treatments, a brow lift might be your best option.

What Is an Endoscopic Brow Lift?

For those who want more than Thermage or Botox can offer but aren't ready for the serious slicing that comes with a full brow lift, an endoscopic brow lift might be an attractive option. In this procedure, the surgeon makes four to six tiny incisions in the scalp, then slips a stainless-steel viewing probe under the skin that allows him or her to pull sagging areas taut and snip the muscles that cause frown lines (but not the muscles that cause horizontal forehead lines); this is a less invasive approach than the conventional brow lift. Although the forehead skin can be lifted somewhat, no excess skin is removed as in a traditional brow lift. The recovery time and postoperative numbness is generally far less with the endoscopic procedure. However, the endoscopic lift tends to be less pronounced, and the results are not nearly as long lasting as with a traditional brow lift. Another potential drawback is that a less experienced surgeon might snip some of the forehead muscles unevenly, resulting in an asymmetrical appearance that could require corrective Botox.

Blepharoplasty (Eyelid Lift)

What it is. As we grow older, the skin of the upper and lower eyelids tends to sag and droop. Our facial fat redistributes around the eyes, first forming small pockets and, as the redistribution progresses, eventually forming bags. This phenomenon is incredibly common, especially in certain families who are genetically predisposed to the condition. The problem is that the excess skin and fat pockets make the eyes look smaller. One of the most commonly performed "invasive" procedures, blepharoplasty (or eyelid surgery) rejuvenates the eyes by removing excess eyelid skin and the bulges of fat appearing on the eyelids; occasionally, it also tightens the muscles beneath the eyes. In some cases, if overhanging upper eyelid skin becomes pronounced enough to interfere with your vision, your health insurance might pay for that part of the procedure

What to expect. Blepharoplasty is performed by plastic surgeons, ocular plastic surgeons (those who specialize in the eyelid), and

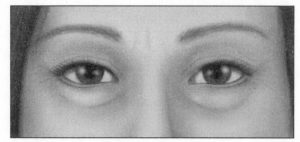

Before blepharoplasty

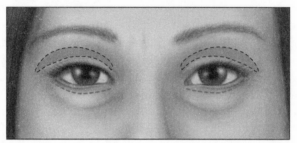

Incision sites and tissue to be removed

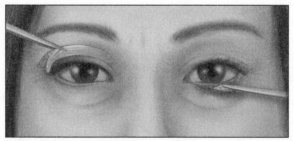

Fat and skin are removed from the outside of the upper lid
Fat is also removed from the inside of the lower lid

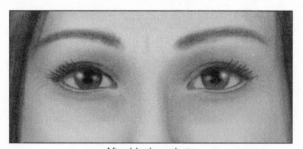

After blepharoplasty

The blepharoplasty procedure.

dermatologic surgeons. They start by numbing the skin around the eyes with a local anesthetic, possibly in combination with a light sedative. (You don't usually have to be put to sleep.) The procedure is divided into two parts: treatment of the upper lids followed by treatment of the lower lids. (Some patients require surgery in one area, whereas others require both.) After making a football-shape, elliptical incision in the crease above the upper eyelid, the surgeon typically remves excess skin, extracts existing pockets of fat, then stitches the skin together. A similar procedure is performed on the lower lid, where the incision is made either just inside the lid or just below it, so that when the wound heals it is hidden from view.

A skilled surgeon will remove just enough skin and fat to achieve a natural-looking result. If too much skin is removed, the lower lid can be pulled down when you open your eye, and you might not be able to close your eyes easily. If too much fat is removed, the pocket under

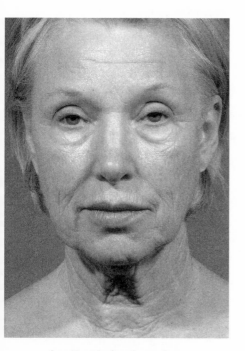

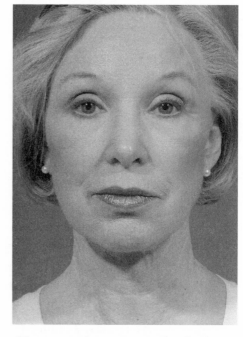

A patient before brow, face, and eyelid-lift surgery.

The same patient seven months after brow, face, and eyelid-lift surgery.

> **Myth**   A face-lift will make my skin tone and texture look younger.
>
> **Truth**   So many of my patients believe this one, and I can't say I blame them. You'd think that a surgical procedure that involved so much expense and recovery time would not only lift the skin but also restore its quality to its original splendor. This is why many people are disappointed to see that the brown spots, dullness, and even some of the crinkles they had before the surgery are still there afterward. However, although a face-lift removes excess skin, it does nothing to help the texture, tone, or quality of the skin. That's why a competent plastic surgeon will either suggest a good skin-care program for you or refer you to a dermatologist, who can use a combination of topical products—along with lasers, peels, Botox, and fillers, if you desire—to clean up the surface of your skin.

the eye will look hollow, which will make you look older, not younger. Once you're stitched up, the scars are usually barely visible. Although you'll almost surely see some bruising and swelling, you'll most likely be back at work and able to resume your regular activities within a week. One of the best aspects of this procedure can also be one of the scariest: since the eyes are truly the windows of the soul, blepharoplasty can change your appearance dramatically. This can be jarring to you and to your loved ones. This is just one more reason to be certain of your decision beforehand, to choose your surgeon very carefully, and to proceed conservatively. You can always have a bit more skin removed if your doctor removes an insufficient amount the first time around, but if too much is removed, it's hard to do anything about it.

Pros. If your eyes appear tired all the time because of excess skin laxity and puffiness, this is a great way to look more refreshed and years younger in a single treatment. Blepharoplasty is much easier than people think. Side effects are rare, and healing takes only about a week.

Cons. The most significant side effects—all extremely rare—are blindness, difficulty closing the eyes, and asymmetrical results. Be sure you find a very experienced, highly skilled surgeon. Less serious side effects include temporary tightening of the lids, swelling, bruising, and eye sensitivity. The biggest myth about blepharoplasty is that it will take care of fine lines and wrinkles around the eyes. In fact, it does next to nothing for them, so you'll have to continue using topicals, and possibly Botox or a laser rejuvenation procedure, to address those. If too much fat is removed, your eye area could end up looking hollowed out, making you look older, not younger. The latest techniques are designed to preserve the volume around the eyes, which helps maintain a youthful fullness.

> **Myth** Liposuction will make my cellulite vanish.
>
> **Truth** I've seen patients spend thousands of dollars trying to eradicate cellulite, so believe me, I *wish* liposuction were a quick fix. Unfortunately, the puckering and dimpling that strikes so many women's thighs and buttocks is due not to too much fat but to the way the female body tends to store and compartmentalize it. This means that suctioning out the fat won't help. In fact, it can make your cellulite more obvious.

Who benefits most. Blepharoplasty is best for people with excess eyelid skin and drooping and puffiness around the eyes. Although Botox might be able to address some of these issues by erasing crow's feet, and fillers can help to soften the tear trough, only blepharoplasty takes care of excess skin and fat around the eyes.

> **Myth** I'm too young to have a face-lift.
>
> **Truth** As with prescription retinoids, Botox, lasers, and fillers, there is no "correct" age at which to have a face-lift or any other cosmetic surgery procedure. Some patients will say to me, "Dr. Dover, I don't mind my sagging neck, but I *hate* the way my eyes look." I know women who love the way they look at sixty, whereas others can't bear to look in the mirror at age forty-five. Whether to undergo any treatment today, next year, or not at all is a very individualized decision that depends on how your face and body are aging and how you feel about your appearance.

> **Myth**   Liposuction is a great method for losing weight.
>
> **Truth**   I've said it before, but it bears repeating: A generally fit woman who has had three children and can't get rid of the bulge in her lower belly, no matter how many Pilates classes she takes, is an excellent candidate for liposuction. Someone who is roughly at her ideal weight but whose saddlebags won't budge despite her excellent eating habits and multiple weekly exercise classes is another. Liposuction is not a weight-loss procedure. When you are overweight, you have excess fat distributed all over your body, not just in a few prime locations. Liposuction is helpful for localized areas of fat that just won't disappear no matter what you do.

Hair Transplantation

What it is. As the name implies, hair transplantation uses the patient's own hair to fill in thinning areas on the scalp or even in the eyebrows. It is usually done for pattern thinning or baldness (the most common type of hair loss in both men and women), but the procedure is also used to refill areas of hair loss due to trauma in, for example, the eyebrow, or in scarring conditions of the scalp where hair has been lost permanently. Many people still associate hair transplantation with those unsightly, Barbie doll–style plugs; however, the treatment has been revolutionized in the past decade. Now individual hairs or a few hairs are transplanted into tiny slits in the scalp so that even I can't always tell a transplant job from the real thing. This remains the best treatment for pronounced hair loss in women.

What to expect. A hair transplant is typically an in-office procedure that is done under local anesthesia, but your doctor might offer you a light sedative. Although there are many ways of carrying out this surgery, here is a classic scenario: Your doctor starts by removing a strip of scalp from an area of the head where the hair is plentiful—generally from the back. Individual hairs and groups of two or three hairs are carefully extracted before transplanting the grafts into very small slits that have been cut in the thinning areas of your scalp. The head is gently cleaned and bandaged after the procedure. Although your new hair usually sheds shortly afterward, it will grow back in a few weeks, assuming that all your grafts take properly. As many as several hundred to a few thousand grafts can be transplanted during a single session. In most instances, several sessions are required to achieve a nice, natural result.

Pros. Hair transplant surgery is a fairly easy, straightforward operation. It is the treatment of choice for pattern baldness in men and women. Since Propecia should not be used by women, and Rogaine produces less than impressive results, hair transplantation is decidedly a woman's best hope for restoring her full, natural mane. The best news is that once the series of procedures is over, your hair will continue to grow forever because the transplanted hair has been taken from a part of your scalp that never goes bald.

Cons. The operation is expensive, tedious, and time-consuming; it usually requires several sessions over a year or two to attain the desired results. Because it involves making numerous and large surgical incisions and hundreds of small slits, the scalp can be tender, swollen, and bruised for several days afterward. Also keep in mind that if your hair is too thin around the back of the head, where doctors usually harvest the hair from, the procedure might not work for you.

Who benefits most. Hair transplantation is best for men and women who are losing their hair because of their age, genetic makeup, or certain medical disorders. It's especially beneficial for women, who often complain that a receding hairline or diffusely thinning hair gives them a masculine appearance. Because hair transplantation has advanced so much in the past several years, we see many patients who want us to replace their unsightly plugs with more natural-looking micrografts. Finally, the procedure offers an excellent way of filling in eyebrows that have been overtweezed or have begun to thin.

Doctor's Orders

Throughout this book, I've stressed the importance of choosing a good doctor: someone who is truly a master in his or her field. This is true whether you're looking for someone to prescribe a retinoid, inject Botox, or treat your brown spots with a laser. It's just as important to choose a doctor wisely if you're going to have cosmetic surgery. I emphasize this point because these procedures are very expensive, and they are almost never covered by insurance. This makes the temptation to base one's choice on cost especially alluring. For example, let's say you're considering a face-lift at age fifty. You're trying to decide between a doctor who is just okay versus one who is superb and charges $3,000 more. If you live until age eighty and spread that $3,000 over thirty years, isn't $100 a year a pittance to pay, especially considering that you have only one face and you probably won't be repeating the procedure again?

Regardless of what surgical procedure you opt for, choose your doctor carefully. Take time to research his or her credentials, check references, and get a referral from a dermatologist, a primary care physician, a respected medical society, or a friend you trust. Be absolutely sure to ask what sort of backup your potential doctor has in case of a medical emergency. You want to shop for quality, not for a good price. It's your face, your body, and your life.

Using Cosmetic Surgery in Tandem with Other Treatments

Not long ago, a new patient walked into my office with brown splotches, wrinkles, and a tired, sagging face. "I know I look terrible," said Anne, age fifty-eight, and she proceeded to ask what creams, lasers, and injectables I had on hand to help her. I was honest with her: although I could certainly refine her skin quality with the tools I had in my office, I wondered aloud whether she had ever considered a face-lift, the only procedure that would significantly tighten her sagging skin. "We can help you to select a highly skilled plastic surgeon," I said, telling her about a face-lift surgeon with whom we work. "Several months later, once you have recovered, we can smooth out your skin and even out the color with laser resurfacing."

At first glance, it might seem as though dermatologists and plastic surgeons are on opposing teams. One side traditionally advocates gradual, minimally invasive approaches, whereas the other side prefers the more dramatic results that come from a few swift incisions with a scalpel. However, any good doctor knows that no one approach is right for everyone; in fact, a combination approach is often just the right tactic for rejuvenating mature skin most completely and most naturally.

This tandem of treatments can be done in any order you wish, as long as you space them apart by several months. If you're still on the fence about which, if any, cosmetic surgery procedures you want—or if you don't have quite the amount of sagging and sun damage that Anne had—you might decide to start with some treatments that seem a little less daunting.

Myth The results of surgical tightening last forever.

Truth Alas, the areas you have tightened, minimized, or otherwise altered don't stay that way forever. After you undergo a face-lift, for example, you'll start to sag again the minute you begin your recovery; that's just the nature of the aging process. The good news is that you'll start to droop from a new baseline, so you'll never end up as saggy as you would have if you had never had a face-lift in the first place. Furthermore, to invoke a familiar refrain, maintaining a good skin-care regimen after your cosmetic surgery procedure will dramatically prolong the life span of your results.

Perhaps you'll begin by cleaning up your skin with a program of good topical skin care. Maybe you'll book a series of intense pulsed light or Fraxel laser treatments to gently even out your complexion's color and tone, or you might want to schedule a nonsurgical skin-tightening procedure such as Thermage to tighten areas that have begun to sag. If you're not fully satisfied with those results, you might then move on to a face-lift, knowing that your skin will look radiant, smooth, and firm once it is done.

Let's say you're sure that you want eyelid surgery, but you also want to smooth away the crinkles and brown spots that are muddling up the area. You can start with an eyelid lift, but since blepharoplasty will do little if anything for superficial skin quality (including fine wrinkles and irregular pigmentation), you might later get a referral for a dermatologist who will prescribe the right batch of creams, fillers, and possible Botox, pigment lasers, or intense pulsed light to knock years off the skin's appearance once the surgery is complete. After all, at the end of the day, all of us—doctors *and* patients—should be on the same team.

Glossary

abdominoplasty This operation is also called a "tummy tuck," but don't be fooled by the cute name. Abdominoplasty is a major surgical procedure that flattens the belly by removing excess fat and skin and tightening the underlying muscles. It is best for individuals who have overhanging skin after weight loss that cannot be treated by liposuction alone.

Accutane The closest we have to a cure for acne, this drug opens pores, dries out the skin by shrinking the sebaceous glands, and probably has some anti-inflammatory benefits as well. Because it comes with potential side effects, ranging from dry skin and chapped lips to depression—and can cause birth defects if you take it while pregnant—the vitamin A derivative is reserved for only the most stubborn, unrelenting cases of acne, including the type of cystic acne that leaves permanent scars.

acne This is a catchall term for the blackheads, whiteheads, papules (red pimples), pustules (pus-filled pimples), and cysts that result when excess sebum and debris clog the pores, attracting bacteria and causing inflammation. Although most people associate the disorder with teenagers, pimples can emerge at any age until menopause, especially during times of hormonal flux. Effective treatments include topicals (like Retin A, benzoyl peroxide, salicylic acid, and antibiotics), oral medications (like antibiotics, birth control pills, other hormones, and Accutane), and various laser and light sources.

alexandrite laser   This is a reliable device for removing hair and unwanted pigment spots like freckles, moles, and brown birthmarks.

alpha hydroxy acid (AHA)   This term includes glycolic, lactic, and fruit acids. Blended into topical lotions and chemical peel solutions, these ingredients break down the uppermost layer of skin cells, increasing cell turnover and revealing brighter, younger-looking skin underneath.

alpha lipoic acid   This is an antioxidant that can help to prevent premature aging of the skin, including the development of fine lines and wrinkles, when it is taken orally or used topically.

antioxidant   By preventing free radicals from damaging and aging healthy skin cells, this ingredient can stave off some aspects of sun-induced skin aging, such as wrinkles and brown spots. It can also potentially reduce the risk of skin cancer. Some of the most promising antioxidants include idebenone (which is in the cream Prevage), coenzyme Q10, vitamins C and E, and botanicals like soy, green tea, malic acid, and pomegranate. Studies show that consuming these ingredients orally might help your skin even more than applying them topically.

Artefill   This filler is made from microspheres of polymethyl methacrylate (or Lucite) suspended in bovine (cow) collagen. The collagen is absorbed by the body after two to four months, leaving behind tiny spherical beads that last forever. This makes Artefill one of the truly permanent fillers.

basal cell carcinoma   The most common type of skin cancer, this develops when the skin's keratinocyte cells reproduce abnormally. It is a very slow-growing skin cancer, most often seen in sun-exposed areas of the body such as the face. It almost never spreads and is almost always cured by surgical excision.

benzoyl peroxide   This popular topical acne fighter works by opening blackheads and whiteheads and killing the bacteria that cause pimples. Although it can be harsh and drying in some skin types, it's the only ingredient I've seen that's been proven to make existing pimples go away. It is especially effective when used with Retin A and a topical or an oral antibiotic.

blepharoplasty   Another name for eyelid lift, and one of the most commonly performed invasive cosmetic procedures, blepharoplasty rejuvenates the eyes by removing the excess skin and sometimes the fat that causes drooping of the upper lids. It also often entails removing the fat, skin, and muscles that form bags beneath the eyes.

blue light therapy   This therapy uses a color and wavelength of light to treat inflammatory acne by killing acne-causing bacteria. It is frequently used in conjunction with Levulan, a topical light-sensitizing medication.

blue reticular leg veins   These are flat, painless leg veins that emerge in a netlike pattern, most often in women with fair skin.

Botox   Approved by the FDA for the treatment of frown lines, Botox is a neuromodulator produced by a type of bacteria that is found virtually everywhere. Dermatologists inject a purified version of this agent in very small, diluted doses to weaken the tiny facial muscles that are responsible for creases and wrinkles caused by repeated negative facial expressions. Botox is also very effective in the treatment of excess sweating.

breast augmentation   This surgical procedure enlarges the size and/or changes the shape of the breasts, usually with implants made of saline, silicone, or, less often, the patient's own fat. Silicone, which had been taken off the American market until recently—some say inappropriately—is now available again. The choice of saline versus silicone implants is best made in consultation with your surgeon.

breast reduction   Also known as reduction mammoplasty, this surgery firms, lightens, and reduces the size of very large breasts by removing fat, skin, and sometimes breast tissue.

brow lift   This surgical procedure helps to rejuvenate the upper face by elevating drooping eyebrows while smoothing the deep lines and furrows in the forehead. (It's also called a forehead lift.) Some patients opt to have a brow lift with a face-lift and/or blepharoplasty (eyelid surgery).

bunny lines   These are tiny creases that form along the sides of the nose. They are especially obvious when you crinkle your nose and tend to worsen with age.

cellulite   Affecting at least 90 percent of women over the age of eighteen in the United States, cellulite appears when the fat just below the skin begins to pucker between the vertical bands of fibrous tissue that contain it. It's usually resistant to exercise and is found even in physically fit women who are at their ideal body weight.

chemical peel   Acid peel solutions are designed to remove the upper layers of the skin's surface and enhance the deeper skin layers. Just how deeply a peel penetrates, and thus how long you need to recover, varies tremendously, from quite superficial to deep, depending on the type of chemical and treatment that you and your doctor choose.

cleanser   Available in sensitive, foamy, granular, creamy, anti-aging, and oil-zapping varieties, these formulas remove excess dirt, debris, and product residue from the skin. This not only makes the complexion look more radiant but also helps any subsequent products you apply to absorb more effectively.

collagen   This protein is a major structural component of the skin, the ligaments, the tendons, and the bones. In the skin, it degrades from years of sun damage and age, resulting in yellowing, wrinkling, and sagging. Since the 1970s, dermatologists have been injecting lips, fine lines, and wrinkles with synthetic collagen derived from cattle, sold under the names Zyderm and Zyplast, a thicker version. In early 2003, the FDA approved two fillers made of human tissue, Cosmoderm and the thicker Cosmoplast. Unlike bovine collagen, the latter two don't cause allergic reactions; thus skin tests prior to treatment are unnecessary.

comedo   A comedo (pl., comedones) is a plug that consists of dead skin cells, oil, and other debris. It forms inside a hair follicle, causing a blackhead (an open comedo) or a whitehead (a closed comedo).

compression sclerotherapy   One of the most popular and effective treatments for big, ropy veins, this variation on traditional sclerotherapy entails wrapping the legs in pressure stockings for two or three days after the injection.

cosmeceutical   This is a hybrid product that straddles the line between a cosmetic and a pharmaceutical prescription.

cosmetic surgery   With an increasing number of minimally invasive treatments available in the dermatologist's office, it's become harder and harder to define just what cosmetic surgery is. Face-lifts and breast augmentation are two obvious examples, but injectable fillers, Botox, and lasers come under this category, too. The last three prove that you don't have to go under the knife, empty your bank account, or spend months of recovery time to see a spectacular change in your appearance.

dermis   Sitting just below the epidermis, this layer of skin is made up of collagen, elastin fibers, hyaluronic acid, hair follicles, sweat glands, and blood vessels.

DMAE   This stands for dimethylaminoethanol, a substance found naturally in fish. Some people believe that it boosts brain power when it is taken orally. Rubbed on topically, it can tighten the skin, at least temporarily.

elastin   This protein gives elasticity to human organs, including the skin. Elastin begins to degrade with age, but other factors, like cigarette smoke, stress, and ultraviolet light, can injure it, leading to premature skin aging.

endoscopic brow lift   In this less invasive alternative to the traditional brow lift, a surgeon makes four to six tiny incisions in the scalp, slips a stainless-steel viewing probe under the skin that will allow him or her to pull sagging areas taut, and sometimes even snips some of the muscles that cause frown lines. The recovery time and postoperative numbness is generally far less with the endoscopic procedure, but the lift tends to be less pronounced and the results shorter-lived.

epidermis   This is the tough, protective outer layer of skin. Its uppermost cells are constantly shedding, bringing new cells to the surface. Its main purpose is to protect the body from external toxins, poisons, germs, and injury.

exfoliant   This is the name for any cleanser or treatment that physically or chemically removes the uppermost layer of skin cells to reveal younger, healthier, and more radiant skin underneath. Scrubs, microdermabrasion, vibradermabrasion, and acid peels all fall into this category.

face-lift   This surgical procedure redrapes the skin to cover the lower part of the face and neck by cutting out excess skin and sometimes fat as well. Less common is the mid-face-lift, which tightens sagging skin in the central portion of the face. Both procedures leave scars and require a healing phase that can range from a few weeks for a minimally invasive face-lift to several weeks for a full face-lift.

filler   A cosmetic filler is a soft material that is injected into unwanted folds, creases, and wrinkles. It makes them invisible until the material is absorbed into the body. Depending on which filler you use, it lasts between three months and virtually forever. Doctors categorize fillers by their ingredients and their longevity. The major temporary fillers consist of collagen, hyaluronic acid, hydroxylapatite, or poly-L-lactic acid. Permanent fillers are made of methyl methacrylate and silicone. Fillers can be used to augment the lip lines and the lips themselves, to fill creases and lines around the mouth, and to address the volume loss that naturally occurs with aging.

fractional lasers This class of lasers, which includes the Fraxel, Fractional CO_2, Active FX, and Profractional, rejuvenates the skin by resurfacing only a fraction of the skin with each treatment, leaving the surrounding areas intact for faster healing and fewer side effects.

GABA This stands for gamma-aminobutyric acid, a neurotransmitter in the body that makes muscles relax. Used topically, the ingredient can help to soften the facial muscles, thus temporarily smoothing the skin.

glabellar creases Also called frown lines, these are deep creases between the eyebrows. They can make you look angry, and they respond beautifully to Botox, used either alone or in conjunction with a soft filler.

growth factor This natural compound is found in young skin cells and in healing wounds. It can be derived from human cells grown in a culture and used as an anti-aging ingredient. Some of the most popular topical growth factor products are TNS Recovery Complex and RéVive.

hair transplantation A procedure that uses the patient's own hair to fill in thinning or bald areas on the scalp. Although many people still associate it with unsightly plugs, the treatment has been revolutionized in the past decade. Individual hairs or clusters of a few hairs are transplanted into tiny slits in the scalp so that even I can't always tell a transplant job from the real thing. Traditionally used for men with thinning scalps, this is a highly effective treatment for hair loss in women as well.

hyaluronic acid   This spongy material is present in the skin's dermis (or second layer). It helps to hold collagen and elastin together, giving the skin support and body. Since it attracts water, hyaluronic acid functions as an excellent moisturizer and temporary skin plumper when it is added to topical lotions and creams. Injected into the skin in the form of highly versatile hyaluronic fillers, like Restylane, Perlane, and Juvederm, it smoothes lines, wrinkles, and creases.

hydroquinone   This drug is used to bleach away freckles, sun-induced brown spots (lentigines), and melasma. It is available in over-the-counter cosmeceuticals as a 2 percent formulation, but it's even more effective in the prescription cream Tri-Luma, which combines a 4 percent hydroquinone solution with Retin-A and a topical steroid. The FDA is considering removing hydroquinone from the market, based on circumstantial evidence that it might be carcinogenic. It has been unavailable in Europe for years.

infrared laser   This includes skin-rejuvenation devices like the Smoothbeam, CoolTouch, and Aramis lasers, which stimulate collagen production, thus helping to improve wrinkled and acne-scarred skin. An infrared laser can also minimize acne by temporarily shrinking the sebaceous glands.

intense pulsed light   This tool is not a laser but rather a device that flashes powerful pulses of broad-spectrum light onto the skin to treat a variety of issues. Intense pulsed light can stimulate collagen production, resulting in smoother, less-wrinkled, younger-looking skin. It can also remove unwanted hair, cause sun-induced brown spots to fade, and reduce redness and facial red blood vessels.

kinetin   A plant-derived hormone found in quite a few cosmeceutical creams, kinetin has long been billed as a nonirritating alternative to retinoids that can help to repair damaged skin cells and protect them from further injury.

KTP laser   This device emits a beam of green light that makes blood vessels invisible and removes sun-induced brown spots from the skin.

It is a great tool for easing facial redness, broken facial blood vessels, flushing, and red birthmarks as well as for evening out skin color from sun damage.

laser   An acronym for "light amplification by stimulated emission of radiation," this class of devices uses a powerful beam of light to selectively alter the skin. Depending on the technique and the wavelength of the light, a laser device can remove hair, decrease the visibility of red vessels, even out pigmentation, smooth wrinkles, or tighten skin. Ablative lasers, which are used to smooth wrinkles and acne scarring, wound the skin to some degree, causing a variable amount of crusting, scabbing, and redness. Nonablative lasers, which are used to decrease skin redness, brown discoloration, and sagging and to remove hair, do not wound the surface of the skin and therefore require little or no healing time.

laser skin resurfacing   This treatment removes much of the skin's wrinkled, scarred, and/or splotchy upper layers, revealing clear, baby-smooth skin underneath. Until recently, the mighty CO_2 was our only option for resurfacing. Although it can make you look at least a decade younger in two weeks, it comes with more than a week of recovery time. Now we have gentler resurfacing devices at our disposal, like the Fraxel, Fractional CO_2, Active FX, Pearl, and the Portrait plasma. All are gentler, often necessitating multiple treatments, but require far less downtime than the traditional CO_2 laser.

LED photomodulation   Light-emitting diodes (LEDs) painlessly stimulate collagen production. After several treatments, some patients notice that their skin looks smoother and creamier, less red, and more even in color, although the changes are usually extremely subtle.

leg-vein stripping   This is a popular surgical procedure for varicose veins that, until very recently, required incisions to be made in the skin at intervals along the length of the vein; small portions of the vein were then extracted. It was usually done under anesthesia and left scars at each incision. Many dermatology offices have replaced this treatment with ambulatory phlebectomy, a less invasive procedure that uses tiny incisions to gently extract small fragments of the vein, or endovenous vein removal, an even less invasive technique in which an ultrasound guided laser or a radio-frequency probe zaps the walls of large veins.

lentigo   This is the medical term for a sun-induced brown spot on the skin. Lentigines accumulate primarily on the face, the hands, the arms, and the legs with age, especially in those who chronically expose themselves to sunlight and tanning beds.

liposuction   This body-sculpting procedure is best for, but not limited to, those who are already close to their ideal weight but have areas of fat that just won't budge. It works best when performed on "love handles," saddlebags, the upper arms, the lower abdomen (below the belly button), the buttocks, the neck, and (for men and even some women) the breasts. Done properly, the outpatient operation removes areas of unwanted fat with minimally invasive techniques and limited anesthesia. Liposuction is not a weight-loss treatment, nor does it cure cellulite.

long-pulsed diode laser   This laser device uses a beam of light to remove hair and reduce the visibility of large facial blue veins and some leg veins. Because of its long pulse duration, it's safer on darker skin types than many other lasers are.

melanoma   The third most common, and by far the most dangerous, form of skin cancer, this results when pigment cells called melanocytes mutate abnormally. Although it's almost 100 percent curable when diagnosed early, it can be fatal if allowed to spread to other parts of the body. About sixty thousand Americans are diagnosed each year with melanoma, resulting in more than eight thousand deaths annually.

melolabial folds   These creases run from the outer corners of the lips to the chin. They are also known as marionette lines.

mesotherapy   Primarily used for fat reduction and the removal of cellulite, this treatment involves the injection of substances that are designed to melt away fat. However, these substances are not regulated, are not approved by the FDA, and have not been properly studied, so patients have no way of knowing how safe or effective they are. The Brazilian government recently banned mesotherapy. This is not an encouraging sign, because Brazil rarely bans anything.

microdermabrasion   This method uses a fine spray of aluminum oxide or salt crystals to gently sandblast the skin, revealing a, brighter, rosier, younger-looking complexion. Microdermabrasion that is administered or supervised by a doctor tends to be (but isn't always) more aggressive than the spa procedures performed by aestheticians.

nasolabial folds   These creases run from the sides of the nose to the mouth and tend to deepen with age.

Nd:YAG laser   A short-pulsed Nd:YAG laser is used to treat lentigines (sun-induced brown spots) and tattoos, whereas the long-pulsed kind is used to remove excess hair in all skin types and to zap unwanted leg veins and blue facial veins.

peptide   Popular in cosmeceuticals, this tiny chain of amino acids can prompt the skin cells to make more collagen, the epidermis to normalize, and the blood vessels to become plumper and healthier—all of which should, in theory, reduce the signs of aging over time. Another emerging class of peptides temporarily relaxes the facial muscles that are responsible for crinkling, so the skin looks smoother and fine lines are less obvious. Copper peptides can cause brown spots to fade and smooth wrinkles very slightly.

photoaging   This is the name for premature aging of the skin caused by exposure to the sun. The symptoms of photoaging include uneven pigmentation, fine lines, and wrinkles.

photodynamic therapy (PDT)   For this combination therapy, which is used to treat acne and the early stages of skin cancer and to rejuvenate maturing skin, dermatologists start by painting a light-sensitive substance called Levulan onto the skin. Then they expose the area to a pulsed dye laser, intense pulsed light, or blue light. Levulan makes these devices far more effective than when they are used alone.

photorejuvenation   This term refers to the use of light and energy sources, like lasers, intense pulsed light, and radio-frequency devices, to reduce or eliminate unwanted pigmentation, fine lines, wrinkles, and sagging areas of the skin.

Portrait plasma   This resurfacing device zaps the skin with a high-energy nitrogen gas, leaving a paper-thin crust that acts as a protective dressing. The treatment can be very gentle, leaving no wound at all and requiring no healing whatsoever, or progressively more aggressive. With more aggressive treatments, once the "dressing" falls off (after a week or so), you're left with a fresh, younger-looking complexion that is smoother and more even in color.

PPX system   Also known as Isolaz, this painless treatment uses gentle suction to open and unclog the pores, clean out sebum, expose the skin to intense pulsed light, reduce skin inflammation, and kill pimple-causing bacteria. The treatment is very effective for blackheads, larger blemishes, and, occasionally, cystic acne. It is also used for hair reduction and photorejuvenation.

pulsed dye laser   This is the first laser that was developed specifically for medical use, about twenty years ago, and it has been improved continually since then. The pulsed dye laser is still the treatment of choice for port-wine stain birthmarks. The latest, enhanced version is also one of the most effective tools we have for treating facial blood vessels, redness, flushing, stretch marks, and scars.

Q-switched laser   This is a highly effective, ultra short-pulsed laser that treats brown spots, birthmarks, and tattoos with minimal discomfort. The alexandrite, ruby, and Nd:YAG are examples of Q-switched lasers that are used in skin treatments.

Radiesse   This thick filler (whose generic name is calcium hydroxyl-apatite) is made from microspheres of a synthetic version of the material found in bones and teeth. Once the spheres are injected, the body slowly produces collagen around them. This filler, which lasts a year or longer, is especially helpful for nasolabial and melolabial folds and for filling hollow cheeks.

red facial blood vessels   These painless veins that become visible along the sides of the nose and cheeks will worsen with age, especially in fair-skinned individuals, but also in those who smoke, consume alcohol regularly, and expose their skin to excessive sun and heat. These vessels are easily treated with a series of pulsed dye laser or KTP laser sessions or with intense pulsed light.

retinoid   This remarkably effective prescription vitamin A derivative helps to shed the cells that make up the outer skin layer, and it replaces them with plumper, healthier ones. Beneath the skin's surface, a retinoid acts to normalize blood vessels and stimulate the production of new collagen fibers and hyaluronic acid. The result is better skin texture, more even color, and increased radiance in as little as two weeks. Prescription products that contain retinoids include Retin-A, Renova, Tazorac, Differin, and Avage.

retinol   A weaker cousin to the retinoid, this nonprescription, over-the-counter ingredient helps to speed cell turnover and possibly generate collagen, making the skin look smoother and more even in color over time.

rosacea   Often mistaken for acne, this disorder is characterized by flushing, broken blood vessels, and later, papules and pustules. The pimples of rosacea respond to topical creams and gels, like MetroGel and Finacea, and to oral antibiotics. However, the redness and the vessels won't get better without laser or light treatments.

sclerotherapy   The treatment of choice for most leg veins, this procedure entails injecting glycerin, saline, or another medical sclerosing agent into visible veins to safely irritate the vessel wall, causing it to collapse and shrivel up.

Sculptra   Made from absorbable suture material, this injectable filler (whose generic name is poly-L-lactic acid) is used for facial contouring and to smooth deep lines, hollows, and depressions. Sculptra stimulates collagen production, so you generally require a minimum of three treatments, spaced one month apart, to see lasting results.

silicone   Used off-label for moderate lines, depressions, creases, and acne scarring, liquid injectable silicone is one of the only truly permanent fillers available.

skin's virtual age (SVA)   Unlike your chronological age, your skin's virtual age refers to the way your complexion looks and feels. Depending on how well you care for your skin, your SVA might be years younger than your actual age, years older, or just about the same.

SmartLipo   This is a trade name for a type of laser lipolysis, a treatment that combines traditional liposuction with a laser that is designed to melt fat and, some believe, tighten the overlying skin. However, the supposed benefits of SmartLipo, which is considerably more expensive than the conventional version, await proof from properly done studies.

SPF   This stands for "sun protection factor" and is followed by a number. The higher the number, the more the sunscreen will shield you from UVB rays, which penetrate the skin and cause tanning, burning, and, in some cases, skin cancer. The SPF does not reflect how well your sunscreen blocks UVA rays, which penetrate more deeply—even through window glass—and cause more of the signs we associate with aging skin, like sallowness and wrinkling, as well as some forms of skin cancer.

spider leg veins   These are tiny red vessels (about the width of a strand of hair) that usually show up on the thighs and upper calves and increase with age. They are best treated with sclerotherapy.

squamous cell carcinoma   A form of skin cancer that develops when keratinocyte cells begin to mutate abnormally. When caught early, these cancers are very treatable with surgical removal. Left untreated, squamous cell carcinoma will metastasize. Squamous cell cancers of the lips and ears are the most worrisome of all.

sunscreen   This lotion, cream, or spray is the single most important anti-aging weapon you can buy. Sunscreen uses chemicals or physical blockers to prevent a certain percentage of ultraviolet light from getting to the skin and attacking and damaging the skin cells. In order to guard against both UVA and UVB, you must wear a sunscreen labeled broad spectrum. Most broad-spectrum sunscreens contain the powerful UVA blocker avobenzone. However, since this ingredient breaks down after exposure to sunlight, some companies are stabilizing it with additives like Dermaplex (used in the Skin Effects line) and Helioplex, which dramatically prolong the life span of the sunscreen. The latest UVA blocker to hit the United States is Mexoryl, which, like Dermaplex and Helioplex, remains stable and effective even after four hours of sunlight exposure.

surfactant   Used to some degree in nearly all soaps and cleansers, surfactants (or detergents) break down and whisk away your skin's natural oils—and with them, dirt and debris. The more surfactants a cleanser has, the better it works. Thus, depending on how sensitive you are to these cleaning ingredients, a high-surfactant formula could irritate your skin and make it blotchy and flaky. In this case, you should look for a lower-surfactant cleanser.

tear trough   The sunken area just beneath the inner corners of the eyes. The skin in this region sags as fat redistributes with age, accentuating shadows and the appearance of dark circles and making the face look tired. Eyelid lifting tightens the skin and removes unwanted fat, but only fillers can soften and smooth out the tear trough.

Thermage   This is a tightening procedure that uses radio frequency to heat the deeper layers of the skin. It tightens sagging areas on the face and the body by remolding and firming up the existing collagen and stimulating collagen production. A single treatment is usually all that is required.

Titan   This infrared light-source device tightens sagging skin by using a deep-heating energy source to remold and tighten collagen below the skin's surface and stimulate new collagen growth over time. A series of three treatments is usually required.

TriActive   This device combines a laser, suction, and localized cooling to help recontour cellulite dimples.

trichloracetic (TCA) peel   This medium-depth peel treats lines and pigmentation. After the treatment, your skin will peel off for about seven days, leaving you raw for a week or two longer. TCA peels are still fairly popular; my practice performs quite a few of them. Generally, they require about a week of downtime. On the upside, a single peel makes a huge difference in the quality of the skin, which is a huge plus for those who don't want to return—or spend the money for—a series of laser or light treatments.

tumescent anesthesia   Considered a safer alternative to general anesthesia for liposuction, this technique uses a local anesthetic diluted with a salt solution. It is injected into the fat before the fat is suctioned out.

ultraviolet light (UV)   These are invisible rays of light that come from the sun (and tanning beds), resulting in worrisome changes in skin cells. The two types that dermatologists are most concerned with are UVB, which penetrates the skin, causing tanning, burning, and possibly skin cancer, and UVA, which penetrates more deeply—even through window glass—causing the signs we associate with aging skin (sallowness and wrinkling) as well as some forms of skin cancer. Only a broad-spectrum sunscreen shields you from both UVA and UVB.

varicose veins   These blue, squishable leg veins can be as thick as an adult pinkie finger when they are engorged with blood. Although they're sometimes painless, they're often associated with leg aches, especially if you've been standing all day. They are best treated with compression sclerotherapy, ambulatory phlebectomy, or an endovenous procedure.

VelaSmooth   This device uses a combination of suction and radio frequency to recontour the dimpling pockets of fat that appear as cellulite. Although it's not a cure, it can be moderately effective in making those pockets less visible and in actual fat reduction.

vibradermabrasion   Like microdermabrasion, this in-office procedure, also known as vibraderm, works by removing layers of dead and damaged skin cells. Because we use textured, gently vibrating paddles to do the job, the resulting redness and swelling are minimal, which makes the procedure an especially good choice for sensitive skin.

Index

abdominoplasty, 226
ablative lasers, 199, 207
Accent, 221
Accutane, 55, 84
  side effects of, 81
acne, 80–84, 209–210
  among adults, 55
  cosmetics and, 89
  cystic, 82, 84, 85, 211, 214
  diet and, 88
  flares, causes of in adults, 81, 82, 84
  inflammatory, 210
  Isolaz PPX system uses for, 211
  laser and light therapy for, 209
  persistent, treatment for, 213–214
  prescription products, borrowing, 81
  product recommendations for, 85–86
  stress and, 88–89, 107
  therapies, starting with mildest, 93
  treatments for, 83–84, 85

acne cosmetica, 89
Active/Deep FX laser, 208
Active FX CO_2 laser, 209
adult acne. *See* acne, among adults
aestheticians, peels performed by, 78
aging
  anti-, weapons for, 26
  early signs of, 1
  fat redistribution and, 176
  functioning of skin during, 22, 24–26, 28
  mirror exercise, and signs of, 160, 228
  moisturizers with benefits for anti-, 75
  options for anti-, *229*
  reversing and preventing signs of, 53, 71
  UV light and, 98
AHA. *See* alpha hydroxy acids
alexandrite lasers, 200, 202, 204, 213

allergic reactions
  to bovine collagen, 174, 179
  to hyaluronic acid filler, 176
  permanent fillers and, 188
  rarity of, 159
  skin tests for, 183. *See also* skin
    tests
  treating, 178
allergy testing, 173. *See also* skin
    tests
alpha hydroxy acids, 17, 63–64
  effect on skin of, 71
  incorporating, 92
  product recommendations for, 64
  using antioxidants in conjunction
    with, 72
ambulatory phlebectomy, 219
antioxidants
  benefits of, 54, 72
  damage-prevention benefits of, 64
  incorporating, 92
  ingesting, 70
  oral, 54, 92
  product recommendations for, 65
  sources for, 70
  sunscreens with, 106, 108
  topical application of, 72, 99
Aramis, 209, 214
Artefill, 188
avobenzone, 98, 104

basal cell carcinoma, 23, 98, 110
benzophenone, 98, 104
benzoyl peroxide, 83, 84, 90
blackheads, 82, 214
  Isolaz PPX system uses for, 211
blepharoplasty, 226
  procedure, *236*

pros and cons, 238–239
  what to expect from, 235,
    237–238
  who benefits most from, 239
blue reticular leg veins, 218
Botox injections, 2, 31, 162–172
  age for starting treatments with,
    168–169
  alternatives to, 171
  background of, 163
  breast lift myths regarding, 228
  calibrating dose of, 165–166
  compared to antiwrinkle creams,
    163
  conditions helped by, 158, 161,
    163, 180
  cost for treatment with, 170–171
  facial areas treated with,
    169–170
  FDA approval for, 163
  for frown lines, before and after
    photographs, *167*
  functioning aspects of, 162–163
  limiting puckering, 25
  as off-label treatments, 158
  possible side effects from,
    163–164
  results of, 166
  re-treatment necessary after, 166
  sites on forehead, *165*
  timing between treatments with,
    166, 168
  tips on areas improved by,
    179–180
  used for excessive sweating, 170
bovine collagen, 174, 183
  allergic reactions to, 179
breast surgery, 226–227

brow lift
  before and after drawings of, *233*
  endoscopic, 235
  pros and cons, 234
  what to expect from, 234
  who benefits most from, 234
brown spots
  approaches to treating, 202
  erasing, with lasers, 91, 201–202
  excessive sun exposure and, 57
  laser treatments of, 211–212
  men's, 199
  reduction of, 77
  staving off, 64, 92
  use of AHAs to help fade, 64
  UV light and, 95
  See also lentigines
buffered peels, 78
Burns, Jay, 232

calcium hydroxylapatite, 187–188
Captique, 184
cellulite, 216–217, 220–221
  creams, 194, 220
  myths regarding liposuction, 239
  resistance to treatments of, 158
chemical exfoliants, 45
chemical peels, 54–55, 77–78, 92
chemical sunscreens,
    recommended, 100–101
cigarette smoke
  avoiding, 25
  free radicals and, 71
  ill effects of, 24, 32
  veins and, 217
cleansers, 26
  answers to quiz on, 37–38
  choosing right, 49

exfoliating, 46, 54. *See also*
    exfoliants
  finding right, 3
  improvements in, 40
  and lowering of SVA, 48–49
  quiz on, 35–37
  recommendations for, 42–44
  skin types and, 41
  spectrum for, 27
  with surfactants, 41
  as treatment staple, 159
cleansing (six-week plan)
  fifties, 134
  forties, 128
  seventies and beyond, 146
  sixties, 140
  thirties, 122–123
  twenties, 117
Clostridium botulinum, 162
CO_2 resurfacing laser, 196–197,
    200, 207, 208, 214
  before and after photographs
    after treatment with, *196*
  recovery time after use of, 197
collagen
  allergic reactions to, 178
  bovine, 174, 179, 183
  derived from pigs, 189
  destruction, 71–72
  fibers, stimulating production of
    new, 53–54, 59–60
  as filler, 157
  human, 174, 183–184
  loss of, 24
  smoking and breakdown of, 32
  speeding up production of, 92–93
  stimulating body to produce,
    186

collagen (*continued*)
  unpredictable regeneration of,
    206
comedones, 82
complexion
  dulling of, 22
  making dramatic change in, 208
  twelve-hour rule and, 57
  understanding SVA of, 3–4
CoolTouch, 209, 214
copper peptides, 67
  product recommendations
    for, 67
  See also peptides
cosmeceuticals
  benefits of, 54
  difference between prescription
    drugs and, 74
  skin-tightening, 24
cosmetic fillers. *See* fillers
cosmetics, acne and, 89
cosmetic surgery
  abdominoplasty, 226
  alternatives to, 200
  answers to quiz on, 225–227
  blepharoplasty, 226, 235–239
  on breasts, 226–227
  brow lift, 233–234
  endoscopic brow lift, 226, 227,
    235
  face-lift, 225
  hair transplantation, 226,
    240–241
  liposuction, 226, 227
  mini-lift, 232
  procedures falling under term,
    229–230
  quiz, 223–225

  using, in tandem with other
    treatments, 242–244
Cosmoderm, 183–184
Cosmoplast, 183–184
creams
  cellulite, 194, 220
  finding right, 3
  skin, versus laser treatments, 208
  See also face creams
creases
  deep, between brows, 159
  effect of Botox on, 163, 169
  glabellar, 58, 168, 171, 189
  sleep-induced, 32
crow's feet, 158
  effect of Botox on, 163, 179
cystic acne, 82, 84, 85, 211, 214

Danby, Bill, 88
dermatologic surgeons
  blepharoplasty performed by, 237
  use of, for Botox procedures,
    164
dermatologists, 28–32
  choosing, 182
  confiding in, 160
  consultations with, 30
  getting information from, about
    fillers, 177
  having suspicious skin spots
    checked by, 110
  for injectables, choosing
    experienced, 162
  locating good, 29–30
  paying attention to advice of,
    31–32
  use of fillers by, 182. *See also*
    fillers

use of, for Botox procedures, 164, 165

using expert, for laser treatments, 199

dermis, 22
    components of, 24
    effect of retinoids on, 59

diet
    acne and, 88
    need for antioxidants in, 112

DMAE (dimethylaminoethanol), 66

doctor, importance of choosing good, 29–30, 227, 238, 241–242

Dysport, 171

eczema, 2

elastin
    loss of, 24
    smoking and breakdown of, 32

Endermologie, 221

endoscopic brow lift, 226, 227, 235

endovenous phlebectomy, 219

enzyme exfoliants, 46

epidermis
    breaking down of, 63
    components of, 22
    effect of retinoids on, 59
    and unbuffered peels, 78
    well-functioning, 23

erbium laser, 200

Evolence, 189

exfoliants, 44–45
    chemical, 45
    enzyme, 46
    how and when to use, 46
    long-term effects of, 37
    physical, 45

product recommendations for, 47–48

eyelid lift. *See* blepharoplasty

face creams, 68, 71
    comparison of Botox to antiwrinkle, 163
    power of, on a fifty-eight-year-old, 139–140
    as treatment staple, 159

face-lift, 225
    before and after drawings of, *231*
    as individualized decision, 239
    problems not corrected by, 238
    pros and cons, 232–233
    as right treatment: Mindy's story, 227–231
    sagging after, 243
    what to expect from, 231
    who benefits most from, 233

facials, 28

fat
    around eyes, gain and loss of, 180
    distribution in women, 220
    loss of, 24, 190
    redistribution of, 176
    reduction devices, 221
    your body's own, used as filler, 185–186
    See also subcutaneous fat

fifties
    cleansing (six-week plan), 134
    prevention (six-week plan), 138
    products for six-week plan, 134, 135, 136, 137, 138, 139
    skin-care regimen for, 133–139
    SVA breakdown, 19–20
    treatment (six-week plan), 135

fillers, 2, 173–190. *See also specific fillers*
  allergic reactions to, 159
  Artefill, 188
  available, 157–158
  bovine collagen, 174
  choosing, 158
  Cosmoderm and Cosmoplast, 183–184
  defining, 174
  European availability of, 180
  Evolence, 189
  finding best, for your needs, 177
  functioning of, 180, 182
  human collagen, 174
  injections with: before and after photographs, *181*
  latest, 161
  life spans of, 177
  liquid injectable silicone, 188–189
  miracle of cosmetic: Deena's story, 172–173
  permanent, 158, 177, 188
  Radiesse, 187–188. *See also* Radiesse
  reference guide: generic and brand names, 175
  replacing lost volume with, 182
  Sculptra, 186–187. *See also* Sculptra
  tips on areas improved by, 179–180
  types of, 183–189
  for under-eye circles, 189–190
  using body's own fat as, 185–186
  volume, 176–180
  working with, as an art form, 182
  Zyderm and Zyplast, 183

Food and Drug Administration (FDA), 54
  -approved botulinum toxin, 171. *See also* Botox injections
  Botox approval by, 163
  Evolence approval by, 189
  first filler approved by, 174
  garnering approval from, 74
  Sculptra approval by, 186
  term *off-label* and, 182
forties
  cleansing (six-week plan), 128
  prevention (six-week plan), 131–132
  products for six-week plan, 128, 129, 130, 131, 132
  skin-care regimen for, 127–132
  SVA breakdown, 19
  treatment (six-week plan), 129
Fractional CO_2 laser, 208, 215
fractional devices, 194, 200, 208–209, 215
Fraxel laser, 208, 215
free radicals, 54, 64
  botanical cosmeceuticals and, 74
  decreasing body's level of, 71
  helping to mop up, 72

GABA (gamma-aminobutyric acid), 66
Gentle Waves light-emitting diodes, 197
glabellar creases, 58, 171, 189
  use of Botox for, 168
glycerin, 71
glycolic acid, 65
  products, lightening pigmentation with, 90

glycolic acid peels, 28, 78
growth factors, 67–69
    benefits of, 74
    lines of, 68–69
    product recommendations for, 69

hair removal
    laser, 194, 200, 204–205
    myths about lasers and
        permanent, 205
    treatment for, 213
hair transplantation, 226
    pros and cons, 241
    what to expect from, 240–241
    who benefits most from, 241
home kits, 79–80
    product recommendations for, 80
human collagen, 174, 183–184
humectants, 71
hyaluronic acid, 184
    derivation of, 178
    enzyme to help break up, 178
    FDA approval for, 176
    as filler, 157–158, 161
    lack of requirement for skin tests
        for, 178
    life span of, 177
    as moisturizing tool, 71
    names of fillers using, 176
    stimulating production of, 53–54,
        59–60
hyaluronidase, 178
hydroquinine, 91
Hylaform, 179
    derivation of, 184
hyperhidrosis, 170

ingredients, decoding lists of, 48

injectables
    answers to questions about,
        157–159
    choosing experienced
        dermatologist for, 162
    expectations for, 161
    increasing availability of, 155
    questions pertaining to, 156–157
    reason for appeal of, 161
in-office treatments, 92–93
    chemical peels, 77–78
    home kit alternatives to, 79–80
    to improve texture, 77
    microdermabrasion, 28, 77, 79,
        92
    preserving results of, 154
    vibradermabrasion, 28, 79, 92
intense pulsed-light devices, 194,
    200, 202, 204, 212, 214
    use on veins of, 217
Isolaz PPX system, 85, 90, 211,
    214

Juvederm, 2, 161, 178, 179
    derivation of, 184
Juvederm Ultra, 176, 182, 184
Juvederm Ultra Plus, 176, 182, 184

keratinocytes, 22
    mutations in, 23
kinetin, 69
    product recommendations for, 69
KTP lasers, 204, 212
    use on veins of, 217

lactic acid, 71
laser, light, and energy sources, 197
    myths regarding, 200

lasers, 85
ablative, 199, 207
alexandrite, 200, 202, 204
cellulite-fighting, 221
common skin issues treated by, 211–215
conditions helped by, 197
differences between, 197
erasing brown spots with, 91, 201–202
erbium, 200
and eye safety, 210
fractional, 194, 200, 208–209
hair removal and, 204–205
helping powers of, 191
and how they work, 195–199
important caveat for, 215
injuries that may be caused by, 198
light sources used in, 195
mid-infrared, 209–210
myths regarding, 216
need for experienced practitioner for, 198
nonablative, 199
red blood vessels and, 202–204
resurfacing, 207–209
ruby, 202, 204, 213
short-pulsed, 202, 212
treatments with, 87
types of, 200, 202
use of, on tanned skin, 99–100
See also laser treatments
laser treatments
aggressive, 197
answers to quiz on, 193–195
choosing right, 211–215
and doctor's experience level, 201

factors influencing outcome of, 200
infrared, 214
with little or no downtime, 197
misconceptions regarding, 193
quiz on, 191–193
versus skin creams, 208
tolerance to Q-switched, 198
using expert dermatologist for, 199
and you, 199–201
See also lasers
leg-vein stripping, 219
lentigines, 196, 200
laser treatments of, 211–212
See also brown spots
light treatments, 194, 214
for acne, 107
need for experienced practitioner for, 198
use of, on tanned skin, 99–100
lines
excessive sun exposure and, 56–57
frown, between eyebrows, 171
of negative facial expression, 163
staving off, 92
use of AHAs to help fade, 64
UV light and, 95
liposuction, 226
excellent candidates for, 240
traditional, 227
long-pulsed diode, 200, 204, 213
lotions
finding right, 3
self-tanning, 99
as treatment staple, 159

Lucite, 188
lycopene, 66, 68

melanoma, 23
    incidence of, 98, 110
    moles and, 111
    treatment for, 111
melasma, 90
melolabial folds, 172, 173, 174,
    176
    softening, 180
    thicker fillers for deep, 182
    use of Evolence for, 189
mesotherapy, cautions against,
    220–221
microdermabrasion, 28, 77, 79, 92
mid-face-lift, 231
mid-infrared lasers, 209–210
mini-lift, 232
moisturizers
    with anti-aging ingredients, 17
    with benefits for anti-aging, 75
    finding right, 3
    good-quality, 54
    product recommendations for,
    76–77
    spiked with haluronic acid, 25–26
    sunscreen, 107, 109
moles, 23
    changes in, 110–111
Myobloc, 171
myths
    about breast lifts, 228
    about drinking lots of water, 18
    about face creams, 68
    about face-lifts, 238, 239
    about facial exercises, 24
    about facials, 28

about lasers, light, and energy
    sources, 195, 200, 216
about liposuction, 239, 240
about long-lasting and permanent
    fillers, 177
about newer cosmetic
    procedures, 227
about sclerotherapy, 219
about self-tanning lotions, 99
about skin-care regimens, 57
about sunglasses, 31
about sunscreens, 103
about surgical tightening, 243
about tanning and acne, 107
about tanning beds, 104
about term off-label, 182
about topical oxygen treatments,
    21
about treatment products, 60

nasolabial folds, 172, 173, 174,
    176
    softening, 180
    thicker fillers for deep, 182
    use of Evolence for, 189
    using fat to add volume to, 186
Nd:YAG lasers, 200, 202, 213
    hair removal and, 204–205
    use on veins of, 217
neuromodulators, 162, 171
New England Journal of Medicine,
    70

occlusives, 71
ocular plastic surgeons, 235
off-label treatments, 158
    meaning of, 182
    using Sculptra, 186

oral supplements, 70, 72
oxygen treatments, 21

PDT. *See* photodynamic therapy (PDT)
Pearl laser, 208, 209, 215
peptides, 65–66
  benefits of, 74
  incorporating, 92
  product recommendations for, 66–67
  See also copper peptides
Perlane, 161, 176, 182
  derivation of, 184
  reactions to, 178
permanent fillers, 158
  complications associated with, 188
  and permanent side effects, 177
pharmeceutical prescriptions, 74
phenol peels, 77
  side effects of, 77–78
photodynamic therapy (PDT), 85, 209, 210, 214
physical exfoliants, 45
physical sunscreens, recommended, 101
pigmentation
  lightening, 90–91
  problems, treatment-induced, 100
  product recommendations for problems involving, 91
  uneven, 57
pimples
  harm from squeezing, 89–90
  Isolaz PPX system uses for, 211
  red or pus-filled, 214
Plasma PSR, 200

plastic surgeon(s), 235
  opinion on mini-lift of, 232
  use of, for Botox procedures, 164
polycystic ovary syndrome, 84
poly-L-lactic acid, 186
polymethyl methacrylate, 188
pore extractions, 28, 211
Portrait plasma energy technology, 208, 209, 215
prescription retinoids
  effects of, 71
  as gold standard, 53–54
  home procedures, 80–84
  and in-office treatments, 77
  lightening pigmentation with, 90
  long-term improvement from, 54
  overuse of, 60
  using antioxidants in conjunction with, 72
  variety of, 61
  See also retinoids
Prevelle, 184
prevention (six-week plan)
  fifties, 138
  forties, 131–132
  seventies and beyond, 150
  sixties, 144
  thirties, 126
  twenties, 120
products for six-week plan
  fifties, 134, 135, 136, 137, 138, 139
  forties, 128, 129, 130, 131, 132
  seventies and beyond, 146, 147, 148, 149, 150
  sixties, 140, 141, 142, 143, 144, 145
  thirties, 123, 124, 125, 126

twenties, 117, 118, 119, 120
Protopic, 178, 179
puckering, 25
pulsed dye lasers, 203, 204, 212, 214
    treating scars with, 213
    use on veins of, 217
Puragen, 184

Q-switched lasers, 194, 198, 200

Radiesse, 161, 176, 177, 187–188
    replacing lost volume with, 180,
        182
red blood vessels, 202–204
    treating facial redness and
        broken, 203–204
ReFirme, 194, 207, 212, 232
Reloxin, 171
Restylane, 2, 161, 173, 176, 182
    derivation of, 184
    reactions to, 178
    treatment, before and after
        photographs, *185*
Retin-A, 60, 159
retinoids, 59–63
    for acne, 83
    best time to apply, 61
    differing concentrations of, 61
    and early signs of skin cancer, 54
    growth factors, as adjuncts to, 69
    hormone billed as alternative to,
        69
    maximizing effectiveness of, 62
    topical, 59. *See also* retinol
    See also prescription retinoids
retinol, 17, 59
    -containing products,
        recommendations for, 62–63

difference between prescription
    retinoids and, 62
See also retinoids
rosacea, 55, 86–87
    product recommendations for,
        87–88
    use of lasers for, 194
ruby lasers, 202, 204, 213

sagging, 216
    after face-lift, 243
    laser treatments and, 212
    main culprit behind facial, 24
    skin, 206–207
scars, treatment of, 213
Sciton MicroLaserPeel, 209, 215
sclerotherapy, 194, 218
    use on leg veins, 217, 219
Sculptra, 161, 176, 177, 186–187
    components of, 186
    FDA approval for, in HIV
        patients, 186
    off-label treatments using, 186
    replacing lost volume with, 180,
        182
sebum, cleaning out, 211
self-tanning sunscreens, 107–108,
    109
seventies and beyond
    cleansing (six-week plan), 146
    prevention (six-week plan),
        150
    products for six-week plan, 146,
        147, 148, 149, 150
    skin-care regimen for, 146–150
    SVA breakdown, 21
    treatment (six-week plan), 147
short-pulsed lasers, 202, 212

silicone
controversy regarding, 158
liquid injectable, 188–189
off-label treatments using, 182
sixties
cleansing (six-week plan), 140
prevention (six-week plan), 144
products for six-week plan, 140,
141, 142, 143, 144, 145
skin-care regimen for, 140–145
SVA breakdown, 20–21
treatment (six-week plan), 141
skin
bacteria growth in, 82
boosting glow and color of, 71
care, key role of good topical, 154
checking, during annual
physicals, 110
cross-section model of, 22
equation for younger-looking, 9
functioning of, during aging, 22,
24–26, 28
having healthy, 112
irritation of, 60
issues, treated by lasers, 211–215
layers of, 22. *See also specific layers*
maintenance, 39
neglect of, 56–57
production, promotion of new, 74
refreshing, after menopause,
145–146
repair time for, 40
sagging, 206–207
texture, treatment for poor,
214–215
-tightening procedures and
cosmeceuticals, 24, 194, 197,
200, 212

treatments, spectrum of, *229*
ultraviolet light's effect on, 102
skin cancer, 23, 98
early detection of, 109–111
excessive sun exposure and, 57
leading cause of, 99
retinoids and early signs of, 54, 60
screening, 28–29
treatment for, 111
skin-care regimen
alpha hydroxy acids, 63–64
antioxidants, 64
best time to start, 57
copper peptides, 67
effectiveness of simple, 159
for a former lifeguard, 126–127
growth factors, 67–69
importance of starting early,
56–57
kinetin, 69
oral supplements, 70
peptides, 65–66
prescribed for a forty-four-year-
old, 132–133
qualities of good, 3
retinoids, 59–63
starting early with, 121–122
surface improvements and, 57–59
three activities of basic, 26
tips for six-week plan, 151–152
upgrading, 59
for your fifties, 133–139
for your forties, 127–132
for your seventies and beyond,
146–150
for your sixties, 140–145
for your thirties, 122–126
for your twenties, 117–120

Skin Effects, 5
skin's virtual age (SVA), 3
    factors determining, 4
    fiftysomething, 19–20
    fortysomething, 19
    quiz, 11–14
    reducing, at age seventy-six,
        150–151
    relation of sun exposure to, 99
    seventysomething and beyond, 21
    six do-at-home steps for lowering,
        32–33, 48–49, 92–93, 111–112
    sixtysomething, 20–21
    thirtysomething, 17–18
    twentysomething, 16–17
skin tests, 176
    essential, 183
    for highly allergic people, 179
    hyaluronic acid and, 178
skin-treatment products
    answers to questions about,
        53–55
    decoding ingredient lists of, 48
    key to finding good, 5–6
    patient awareness of, 2
    questions pertaining to, 51–52
sleep wrinkles, 32
S-lift, 232
SmartLipo, 227
Smoothbeam, 209, 214
Sotradecol, 217
SPF (sun protection factor)
        number, 98, *102*
    calculations for, 103
    formulas with high, 103
spider leg veins, 218
squamous cell carcinoma, 23, 98,
    110

stress, acne and, 88–89, 107
StriVectin, 163
subcutaneous fat, 22, 24–25
sun exposure
    aging caused by, 102
    delayed effects of, 17
    excessive, 23, 25, 56–57. *See also*
        skin cancer
    skin's virtual age (SVA) and,
        99
    treatment for cumulative, 214
    ways to avoid, 105
    while driving, 18
    in a young woman, 55–56
sunglasses, 31
sun protection
    answers to quiz on, 97–99
    clothing lines for, 106
    measures for, 97
    need for, 95
    practicing good, 215
    quiz to measure, 96–97
sunscreen, 26
    agents necessary in, 98
    application of, 105, 111
    benefits of good, 102
    broad spectrum, 104
    choosing, *102*
    importance of using, 54, 56, 92,
        98
    reading labels on, 112
    recommendations for, 100–101,
        106–109
    self-tanning lotions and need
        for, 99
    SPF number in, 98, 103
    types of, 104
superficial peels, 78

SVA. *See* skin's virtual age (SVA)
sweating, excessive, 170

tanning lotions, 98
  self-, myth regarding, 99
tanning salons, 95, 99
  curbing addiction to, 108
  damage caused by, 104
  UV light in, 97, 104
Thermage, 194, 197, 200, 206–207,
    212, 232, 233
thirties
  cleansing (six-week plan),
    122–123
  prevention (six-week plan), 126
  products for six-week plan, 123,
    124, 125, 126
  skin-care regimen for, 122–126
  SVA breakdown, 17–18
  treatment (six-week plan),
    124–125
tightening devices, 194, 206
  new, 207
Titan, 194, 207, 212, 232
titanium dioxide, 104
topical products
  beyond, 153–154
  power of, 72–73, 75
treatment plans, 70
  to look younger in four to six
    weeks, 71
  to look younger in three months
    and beyond, 71–72
  to look younger tomorrow
    morning, 71
treatment (six-week plan)
  fifties, 135
  forties, 129

seventies and beyond, 147
sixties, 141
thirties, 124–125
twenties, 118
TriActive, 221
trichloracetic acid (TCA) peels,
    78
twelve-hour rule
  and complexion, 57
  heeding, 92
twenties
  cleansing (six-week plan), 117
  prevention (six-week plan), 120
  products for six-week plan, 117,
    118, 119, 120
  skin-care regimen for, 117–120
  SVA breakdown, 16–17
  treatment (six-week plan), 118

ultraviolet light, 54
  absorption and blockage of, 98
  antioxidants as added protection
    from, 99
  curbing addiction to, 108
  free radicals and, 71
  shielding skin from, 95
  in tanning salons, 97
  two main types of, 102
  and visible aging of face, 98
unbuffered peels, 78
UVA
  guarding against, 104
  rays, 98
  skin penetration by, 102
  sunscreen agents, 98
UVB
  guarding against, 104
  rays, 98

screening, 103
skin penetration by, 102
sunscreen agents, 98
UV light. *See* ultraviolet light

varicose veins, 218
alternative treatment for, 219
treatment for, 218–219
veins, 216–217
blue reticular leg, 218
collapsing of, 217
spider leg, 218
treatments for, 217
varicose, 218–219
VelaSmooth, 221
vibradermabrasion, 28, 79, 92
volume fillers, 176–180

water, 18
whiteheads, 82, 214
harm from squeezing, 89–90
Isolaz PPX system uses for, 211
Willett, Walter, 70
wrinkles
effect of Botox on, 163
long-term prevention of, 17
reduction of deep, 77
staving off, 64
sunscreens for smoothing, 106,
108
UV light and, 95

zinc oxide, 98, 104
Zyderm, 183
Zyplast, 183